THE COMPLETE BOOK OF LUK PRA KOB & HERBAL BALLS

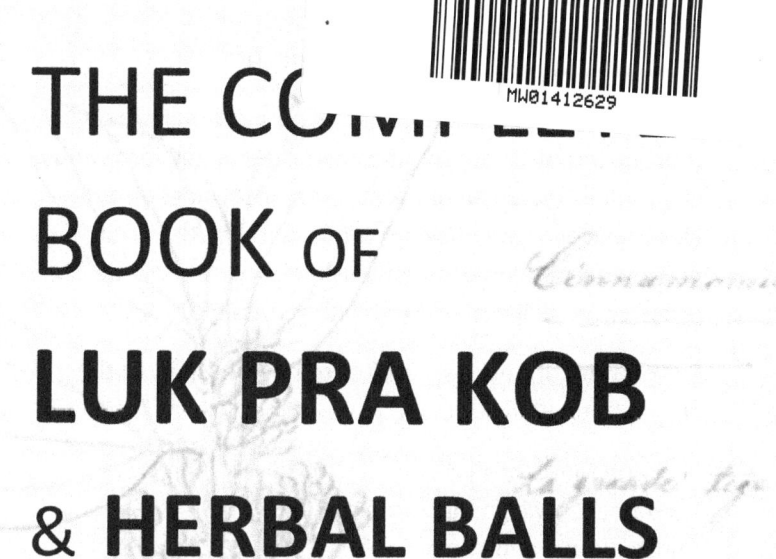

BY **ELEFTERIA** MANTZOROU

Copyright © 2018 by Eleftheria Mantzorou.

All rights reserved. No part of this publication may be reproduced, distributed, or transmitted in any form or by any means, including photocopying, recording, or other electronic or mechanical methods, without the prior written permission of the publisher. Violators will be prosecuted to the maximum extent possible.

For permission requests, write to the publisher, at the address below.

Elefteria Mantzorou
Flow.heavenly@gmail.com
Jointheflow.weebly.com

Although the author and publisher have made every effort to ensure that the information in this book was correct at press time, the author and publisher do not assume and hereby disclaim any liability to any party for any loss, damage, or disruption caused by errors or omissions, whether such errors or omissions result from negligence, accident, or any other cause.

This book is not intended as a substitute for the medical advice of physicians. The reader should regularly consult a physician in matters relating to his/her health and particularly with respect to any symptoms that may require diagnosis or medical attention.

Contents

Introduction 7
What is Luk Pra Kob 8
How herbal balls work 10
The tradition of *Luk Pra Kob* and herbal medicine in Thailand 11
Benefits of Herbal Ball treatment 15
Contraindications & precautions 17
Equipment 18
    Choosing a steamer 19
        Simple rules for safe steaming 22
    The right type of fabric 24
    Strings 26
Luk Pra Kob and Yam Khang 28
The Thai herbs 34
    Eucalyptus 35
    Phlai ginger 37
    Camphor 40
    Kaffir lime 42
    Thai mint 44
    Turmeric 46
    Lemongrass 49
    Tamarind 51
    Cumin 53
    Jasmine 54
Thai herbs generally hard to find in the West 55

Cinnamon leaf 56

　　Alpinia galanga 58

　　Zerumbet ginger (Zingiber zerumbet) 63

　　Blumea balsamifera 64

　　Cardamoms 65

　　Other herbs 65

Making herbal balls with Western herbs 66

　　Lemon 67

　　Ginger 69

　　Calendula 72

　　Lavender 73

　　Chamomile 74

　　Mallow 75

　　Lemon balm 76

　　Willow 77

　　Comfrey 78

　　Other Western herbs for packs and poultices 79

　　A note on Western poultices 79

Using sand, salt, stones and rice 81

　　Using sand 81

　　Using salt 82

　　Using stones and pebbles 83

　　Adding rice in the packs 84

Preparation of herbal balls 85

Methods of tying 89

　　Method #1 – Lazy Girl's Compress 90

　　Method #2 – Easy & Elegant 93

- Method #3 – The Rose Bud 96
- Method #4 – The Thai Way 100
- Recipes 105
- Applications in massage therapy 113
  - Using packs in Swedish Massage 114
  - Using herbal packs in Thai Massage 117
    - Techniques 117
- Lay-outs & protocols 119
  - Lower back pain & sciatica 120
  - Neck tension & upper back pain 122
  - Epicondylitis 124
  - Headaches 126
  - Emotional stress 128
  - Knee pain 129
  - Dysmenorrhea 131
  - Chronic breathing disorders 132
  - Common cold & flu 133
- Sip Sen – The Ten Lines 135
  - 1, 2. Itha & Pingkala sen 137
  - 3. Sumana Sen 139
  - 4. Kalatharee Sen 140
  - 5, 6. Sahatsarangsi & Tawaree Sen 142
  - 7. Nantakawat Sen 143
  - 8, 9. Lawusang & Ulanga Sen 144
  - 10. Kitcha Sen 145
- Foraging for herbs 147
- How to store herbs and herbal balls 149

Epilogue	151
About the author	152
Other works	154
Credits	157
References	158

Introduction

I am very glad I finally got to write this book! During my (many!) years as a massage therapist and instructor, I have not found another thermal treatment as effective as the one that consists of hot herbal balls.

I had the unique luck to learn this art in Thailand, by the late Mama Lek Chaiya, and her son Jack, in 2002. Since then, I have performed hundreds, maybe thousands of treatments with herbal balls (or luk pra kob, as they are known in Thailand).

Having done extensive studies on herbal medicine and aromatherapy, I was able to substitute some of the hard-to-find Thai herbs. However, most of the herbs I use in the balls are included in the Thai recipes.

In this book, I am presenting both the Thai herbs that are used in the compresses, and some Western ones, which can be found easily and have decent medicinal properties. We'll also see how to make and use these herbal balls.

I hope that this book will inspire you to make your own herbal balls, either for your work or for your friends and family. Making herbal balls is easy, effective and fragrant!

What is Luk Pra Kob

Technically speaking, herbal balls are poultices. In the language of herbal medicine, a poultice (also called a cataplasm) is a soft moist mass which may consist of herbs, cereals, clay, salt or minerals, and is spread on cloth over the skin to treat an aching, inflamed or painful part of the body.

In this book, we will speak about the beautiful poultices that resemble a ball. However, feel free to incorporate these recipes in a simply tied and applied poultice, for home and family use.

In Thailand, herbal balls (also known as "compress", "bolus" or "packs") are called Luk Pra Kob – i.e. "pressure with a ball that contains plants". In this book, the words "ball", "packs", "compresses" and "poultices" are synonyms.

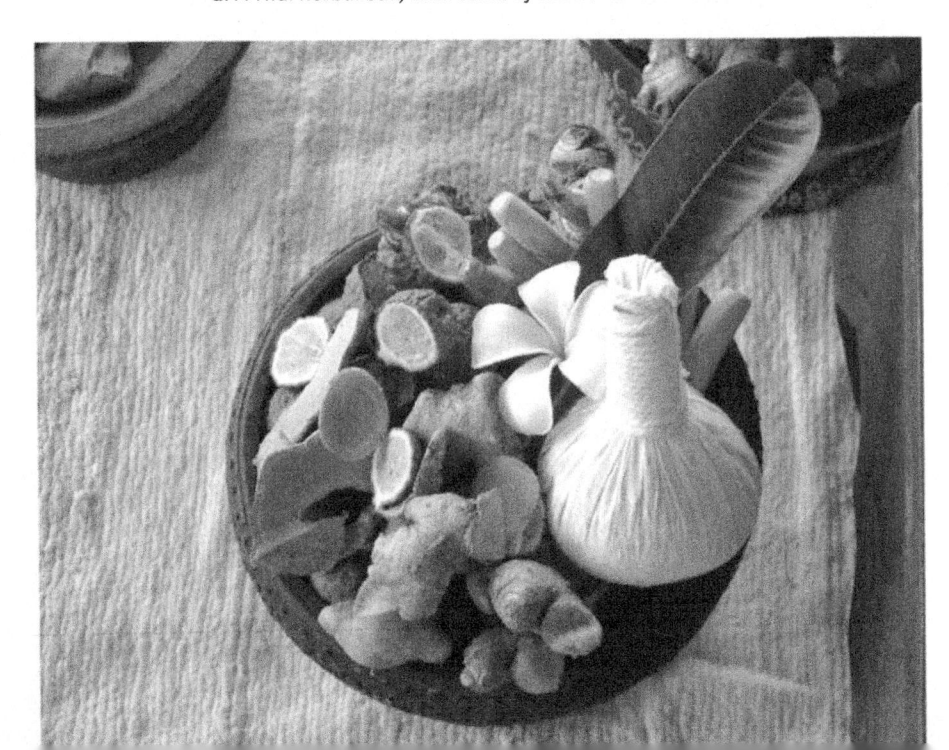

1. A Thai herbal ball, with some of the herbs it contains.

The balls consist of a combination of medicinal herbs, which are placed in a piece of cloth. These compresses are then steam-heated and placed directly on the skin.

Making these balls is easy and cost-effective. Many of the herbs can be foraged, and those that are not available in the wild, are cheap and readily available. Moreover, it takes very little time to prepare an herbal ball, and the process is not messy. You probably have already the tools needed (scissors and knife), and steamers are easy to find (and they are inexpensive!).

The fragrance from the thermal application of the herbal balls will linger in your space for days, and so far I have not met anyone who does not LOVE it!

Herbal packs can be used in many settings, including luxury spas and massage therapy offices, and of course in your home!

How herbal balls work

The effectiveness of the herbal balls is achieved mainly thanks to *thermal conduction*. This term pertains to the transfer of thermal energy by the collisions of microscopic particles and movement of electrons within a body.

Heat spontaneously flows from a hotter to a colder body. For example, heat is conducted from the hotplate of an electric stove to the bottom of a saucepan in contact with it. In our case, the heat from the herbal balls is transferred to the human body, which will be always colder than a steamed herbal ball.

The heat dilates blood vessels and increases topically the blood flow. This relieves pain and swelling. Moist heat is also good for respiratory issues, as it decongests and soothes nasal passages and bronchi.

This heat of course, is not plain steam. It is enriched with the medicinal compounds of the herbs. Moreover, the steam opens the pores of the skin, thus allowing the beneficial compounds to reach deep layers of the body.

As we will see in the section that discusses the medicinal properties of the herbs that are suitable for the application of Luk Pra Kob, most of these compounds have a potent anti-inflammatory effect.

The tradition of *Luk Pra Kob* and herbal medicine in Thailand

Thailand has an autonomous medical tradition, the traditional Thai (or T'ai) Medicine. This tradition has been shaped and influenced by many factors, during a development that lasted many centuries:

- Pre-history indigenous regional practices with a strong animistic foundation.
- Animistic traditions of the Mon and Khmer peoples who occupied the region prior to the migration of the T'ai peoples.
- T'ai medicine itself, as it was developed in the Royal court.
- Indian medical knowledge coming through the Mon-Khmer civilization, which was very powerful in the region, when the Tai people arrived [i]. The Mon-Khmer civilization was heavily influenced by Indian culture, and the Tai people adopted and adapted their indianized culture, when they conquered them [1]. Hence the influence of Ayurveda in Thai traditional medicine.
- Buddhist medical knowledge via the Mon peoples. Moreover, Buddhism became the national religion of Thailand.
- Chinese medical knowledge with the migration of the T'ais who came largely from southern China, and later from the migration of Chinese people in Thailand.

---

[1] This occurs often throughout history. The Romans adopted the Greek culture when they conquered them, and Kublai Khan adopted many Chinese ideals.

In Northern Thailand, especially in Chiang Mai, Lanna medicine – a regional form of local, indigenous medicine – was developed alongside the "official" medicine of the Royal Court.. Many Lanna traditions are still alive, and possibly reflect the most preserved form of the roots of Thai medicine. Herbalism – and animism – play an important role in the medical tradition of Northern Thailand, both in urban and rural environments.

2. Statue of Jivaka in Chiang Mai. Being Buddha's personal physician, Jivaka is regarded as the "father of medicine" in Thailand.

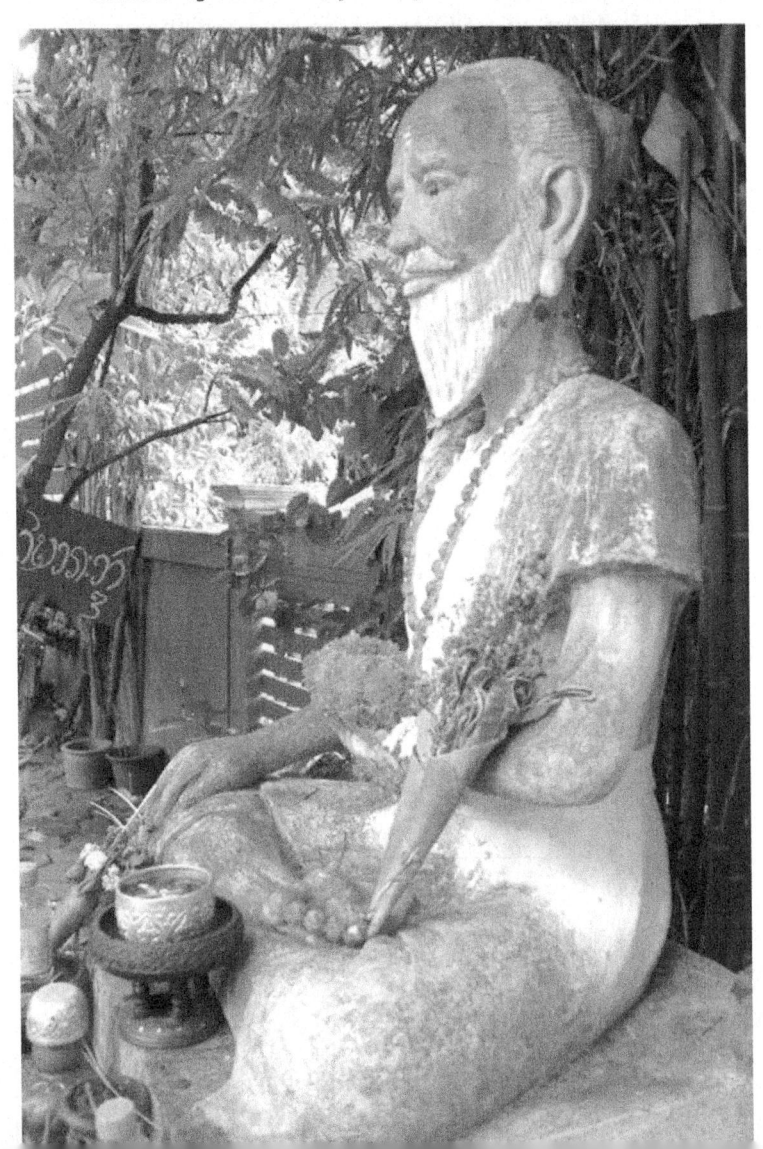

Thai people use a large variety of herbs, both internally and externally. The internal use pertains to the Thai diet and cuisine, which employs a great array of aromatic herbs and spices (I'm telling you, it's delicious!) and to the oral administration of herbs for various health problems.

Of course, herbs are applied externally, quite extensively, through balms and….yes, herbal balls and compresses! This is called "Herbal Massage" in Thailand, and it is very popular. It is usually applied during Thai massage treatments.

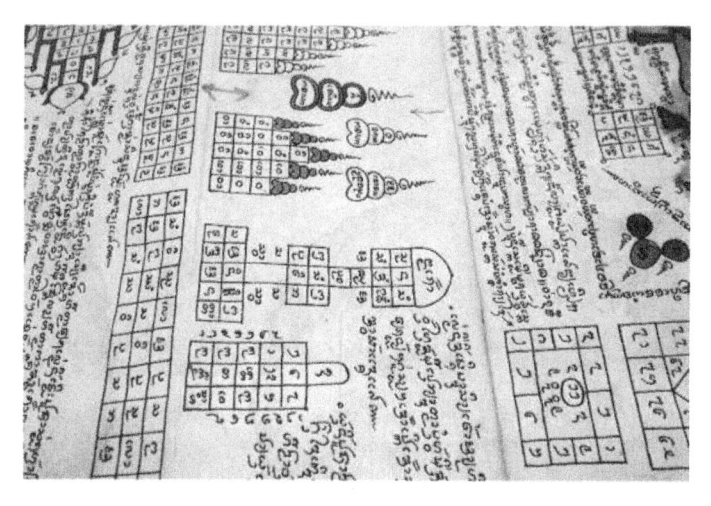

3. Traditional Thai medical manuscripts that reflect Lanna animistic practices. These are symbols for protection, and many of them are used in tattoos. Photo taken in Hang Dong Thai Massage School, by Elefteria Mantzorou.

Herbal balls are part of Ayurvedic treatments as well, where herbs are chosen according to the *dosha* (constitution) of the patient. Although the *tridosha* concept exists in Thai medicine as well, I have never seen a Thai therapist examining the pulse or the tongue of a patient (as is the case in Ayurveda) before treating him/her with herbal balls. The recipe is either standard, or it is formulated according to the musculoskeletal or respiratory issues the patient will mention.

In any case, most of the herbs that are added in the compresses, possess anti-inflammatory properties or valuable aromatic compounds.

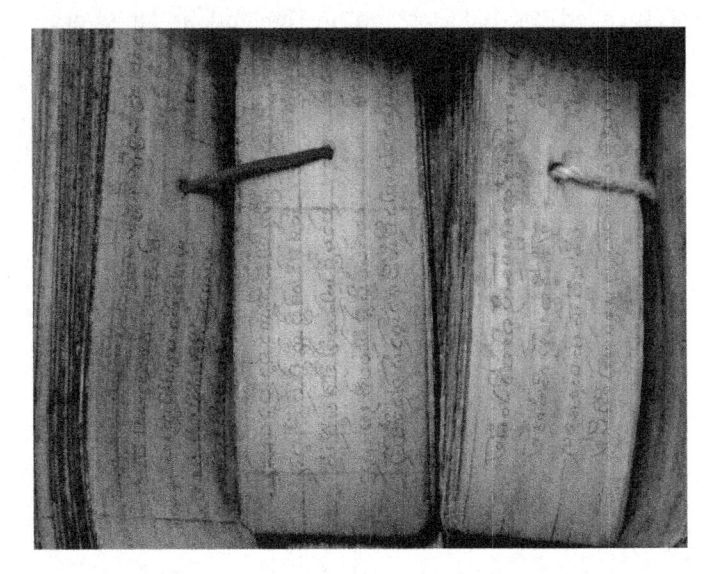

4. Thai medical palm-leaf manuscripts. Palm leaves were used as writing materials in Southeast Asia dating back to the 5th century BCE [ii] and possibly much earlier. The palm leaves are first cooked and dried. The writer then uses a knife pen to inscribe letters. Photo taken in Hang Dong Thai Massage School, by Elefteria Mantzorou.

Most of the herbs that are used in the herbal balls, are also used in Thai balms, which are a very valuable tool, both for the professional massage therapist, and for the general population. The most important herbs are phlai ginger and camphor (ka-boom).

Benefits of Herbal Ball treatment

Most typical Thai recipes for herbal packs are mainly indicated for problems of the musculoskeletal system. This is because most of the herbs have potent anti-inflammatory properties.

Thus, they can be used for chronic injuries or pain:

- Joint and ligament pain – e.g. knee pain (especially pain that is due to osteoarthritis), carpal tunnel syndrome, epicondylitis etc.
- Muscle aches and stiffness – e.g. lower back pain, upper back pain, leg pain.
- Nerve pain and compression – e.g. sciatica.
- Inflammation and chronic injuries of the tendons – e.g. supraspinatus pain.

They are also very effective for respiratory problems, both acute and chronic.

- Use them for asthma and bronchitis.
- Useful for sinusitis.
- Very effective for the common cold and the flu.

They also have the following additional applications:

- Thanks to the aroma and the heat, herbal packs are also beneficial during stressful times.
- If placed on the correct spots, they can be useful for dysmenorrhea (their effect is analgesic anyway). [iii]
- Placed on the head and some special acupressure spots, they can be quite effective for headaches.

- They can be used for insufficient and / or delayed lactation[iv]. I have never seen this application in Europe, although it is well documented in Thai studies. It has even been used in post cesarean and postpartum mothers who had no milk production within 2 hours after delivery. In some cases, the application of herbal compress was accompanied by breast massage. [v]
- In Thailand, warm herbal balls are also used for labor pain – especially for the relief of early postpartum backache. [vi]

5. Thai herbs, ready to be cut and added in compresses.

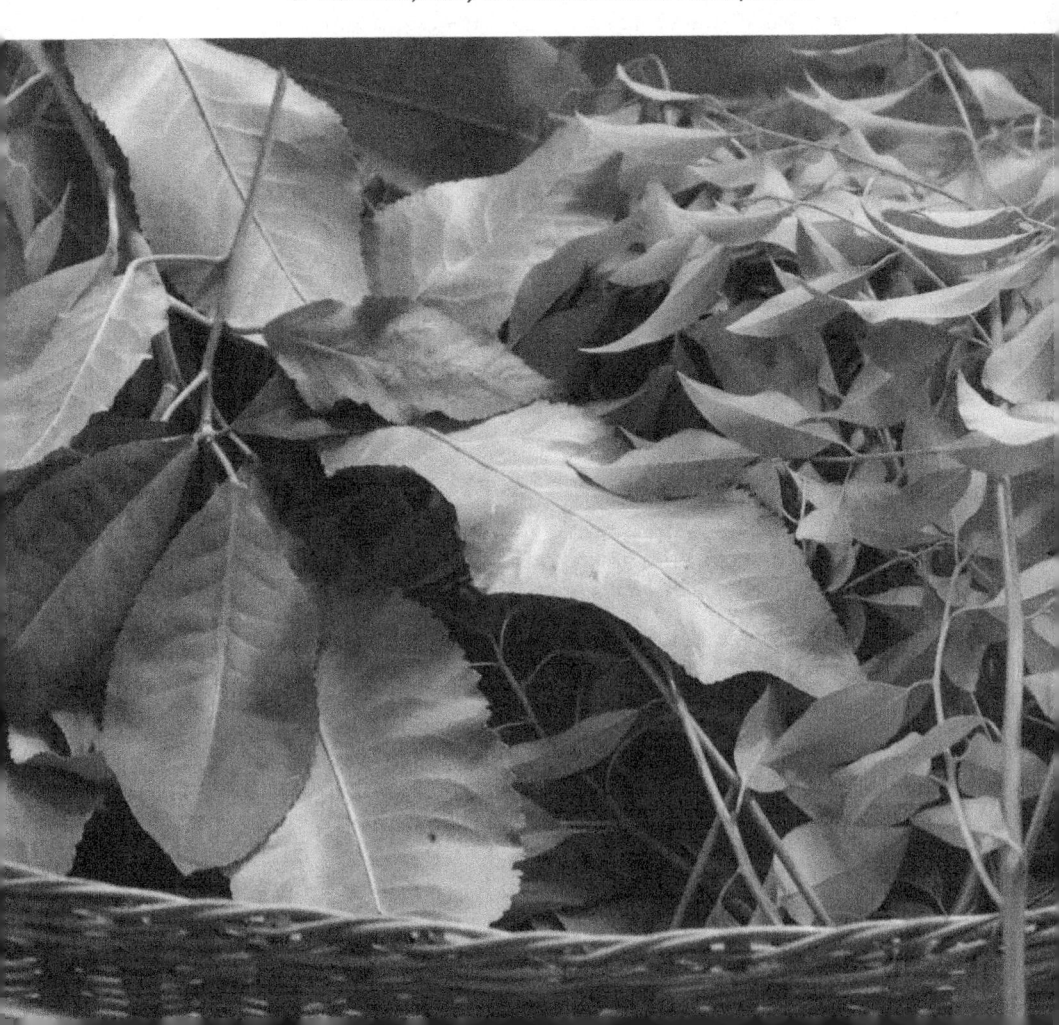

Contraindications & precautions

Herbal ball treatment is generally safe. However, keep in mind the following precautions.

- Herbal packs are a thermal treatment, and like most thermal treatments, it is contraindicated during pregnancy.
- Heat should not be used for the first 48 hours after an injury, as it brings more blood to the area where it is applied. Use cold packs instead.
- Do not place hot packs on eczema, broken capillaries and wounds.
- Camphor and peppermint may not be suitable for people with G6PD deficiency.
- Camphor is not suitable for kids.
- Have in mind that the effect of an herb on the skin can be very different than that which follows ingestion. Never assume that an herb which can be used externally is also safe to be taken as a tea, and vice versa.
- Mind the heat! If a poultice is too hot for your hand, it will be too hot for the client's body, and may cause a burn.
- Remember: the lumbar area is very sensitive to heat. A poultice that be comfortably warm for the neck, can be unbearable for the lumbar area.
- Some herbs (especially turmeric and eucalyptus) may leave permanent stains on fabric.

Equipment

So here's what you will need for the herbal balls:

- 2 pieces of white cotton, hemp or linen fabric, 50 cm X 50 cm.
- 2 pieces of undyed cotton, yucca or hemp string, about 50 cm each, for tying the herbal ball. This is actually optional, since it is possible to tie it with a stripe of the cloth you are using for the balls (refer to the section "Methods of tying").
- The herbs you will use for your recipe (refer to the section "Recipes").
- One medium-sized thick towel. It is best if it is dark green or black, so that the stains from the herbs are not visible after your treatments.
- One steamer. It is possible to use a specialized herbal poultice steamer, or even a bamboo or rice steamer.

Of course, you will also need a massage table, massage oil, or a Thai mat, if you are using the herbal balls during a treatment. What I list above are just the materials you will need in order to make and heat the poultices.

Choosing a steamer

The herbal balls should be heated in steam. They should never be boiled or immersed in water, because they will lose their therapeutic value. Steaming ensures that they retain their medicinal compounds.

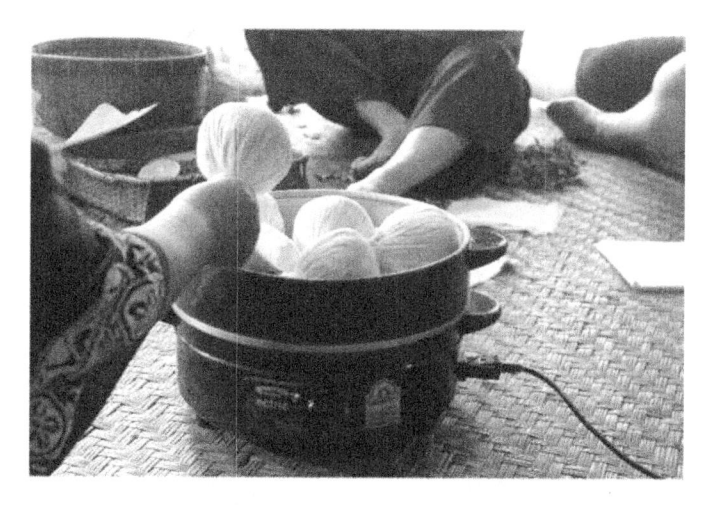

6. Preparing herbal balls for steaming in Chiang Mai, in an electric steamer made of stainless steel.

Steamers come in two varieties: electric or stovetop. Although it is possible to use a stovetop steamer, it is definitely more convenient to use an electric one. Electric steamers can be made of stainless steel or plastic. Both have advantages and disadvantages.

First of all, all steamers have a perforated tray, which allows the steam to pass through a chamber and heat the material that is placed in the "cooker". Yes, that's right, in the cooker! Which means you can use an inexpensive food steamer, and not a perhaps more expensive appliance that is designated especially for herbal treatments.

A steamer made from stainless steel will be sturdier, for sure. However, it has two disadvantages: The first is that it is heavier, and thus inconvenient for the mobile therapist. The second disadvantage is that you will not be able to see the herbal balls being steamed, which is a nice thing to see of course!

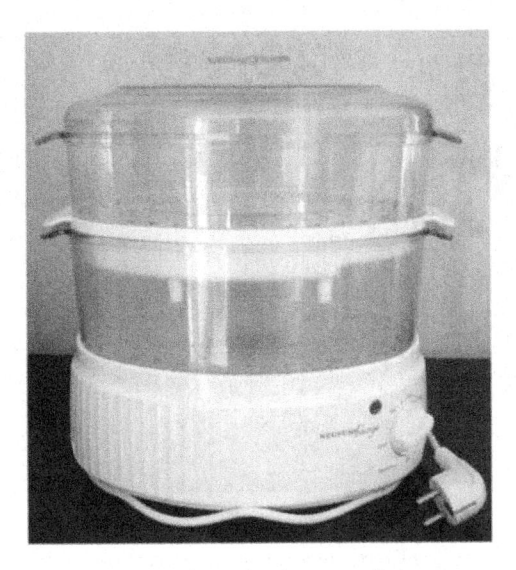

7. A plastic food steamer[vii].

A steamer made from plastic will be lighter and easier to carry. It will also allow you the visual experience of watching the compresses being steamed. However, plastic is not good for the environment, and if it contains BPA it is not good for your health either. In fact, nowadays most commercially available plastic food steamers are BPA-free – look for these ones.

There are some glass steamers as well, but I do not recommend them. The reason is that they may break, and you just don't want that to happen during a professional massage session. However, if you do have a glass steamer and you just wish to use herbal balls to your family members or friends, go ahead and do it.

In Thailand, most therapists and spas use stainless steel steamers.

Now let's have a look at the stovetop options. Stovetop steamers are actually accessories that are meant to fit in various cooking pots. Pressure cooker accessories, like steamer baskets, trays and racks are absolutely suitable. Bamboo baskets can also be used.

An interesting insert is the so-called flower-style steamer, whose perforated "petals" unfold in the pot. This type of steamer baskets is available in silicone and stainless steel, and both types are suitable for herbal ball steaming. These inserts can be fitted easily in any pot, and placed on a small portable gas stove. I have actually worked with this as a mobile therapist, and it can be quite convenient, considering the fact that you do not need a plug nearby, and that you are not consuming electricity in the client's space.

 I do not recommend you to buy any stovetop insert – just use them if you already have them. A light electric steamer is by far the best solution for the professional application of herbal ball therapy.

I am aware of the fact that some therapists are using a microwave oven in order to heat their herbal balls, but I consider that inappropriate.

Simple rules for safe steaming

A few things to keep in mind for safe steaming:

- When you open the steamer, open the lid away from your face and hands—the hot steam can cause burns.
- When you remove the hot herbal balls from the steamer, be careful not to touch the steaming rack, because this will cause a burn. In the beginning, you can use tongs. When you familiarize yourself with the temperature and the whole process, tongs will not be necessary. In fact, I have never used them, although I know some people who do find them useful.
- Be sure to add enough water (more is better!) to the steamer so that it will last through the entire time of your treatment. Set the timer according to the estimated duration of your treatment, or a bit longer. Some steamers have a "keep warm" setting, although I have worked very satisfactorily with appliances which did not have this setting.
- Remember that if you need to add more water, the temperature will drop, and your herbal balls will be a bit cooler for a while. However, if they have been thoroughly steamed for at least 20 minutes, they will be adequately reheated in a few seconds.
- In all electric steamers, the water reservoir can be filled and replenished externally, and a window lets you monitor when the water is getting low. Of course, you do not want to interrupt your treatment in order to replenish the water, so I'll repeat: Be sure to add enough water in the steamer in the beginning of your treatment. In

case you make a wrong estimation, be sure to have some extra water in a pot, in your treatment room (especially recommended for beginners)!
- If you are using a stovetop steamer, be sure that your pot is not boiling dry, which will scorch the pot and could damage it. This is one more advantage of electric steamers: most will stop functioning automatically if they run out of water.

Fun fact

Human beings have been using steamers in order to prepare food and medicine from the depths of antiquity. Some of the world's earliest examples of steam cooking were found in Gunma Prefecture, Japan. They were created during the Stone Age.

Some of the second earliest examples of steam cooking have been found in Italy and Sardinia, created during the Bronze Age, and in Cochise County, Arizona, where steam pits were used for cooking about 10,000 years ago.

In China's Yellow River Valley, early steam cookers made of stoneware have been found dating back as far as 5,000 BCE. They were used mainly to cook rice [viii].

The right type of fabric

I recommend a fabric made from natural fibers for your herbal balls. Suitable types of fibers include:

- Cotton
- Linen
- Hemp
- Silk (not suitable for vegans).
- Bamboo

The fabric has to be white. If it is colored, the colors may bleed when exposed to the steam, and drip on your sheets, and possibly on the client's body or clothes! We're talking about a disaster…

The only type of colored fabric which will not bleed when exposed to steam, is fabric for bed sheets. This type of fabric is made to survive washing in high temperatures. However, I still would not risk it. I always use white fabric for my herbal balls, to be on the safe side.

Fabric density is also an important factor. If the fabric is too thick, the medicinal compounds of the herbs will not be transferred to the client's body as they should. Moreover, you will not be able to roll and tie the herbal ball properly. On the other hand, if the fabric is too loose, some plant particles will slip through from the herbal ball and end up… God knows where. I don't even want to imagine what could happen if some plant material would leak from a compress placed on the lower lumbar region.

I would say that a fabric of 50 denier is a decent choice (denier is a unit of measurement that expresses fiber thickness of individual threads or filaments in fabric or textiles).

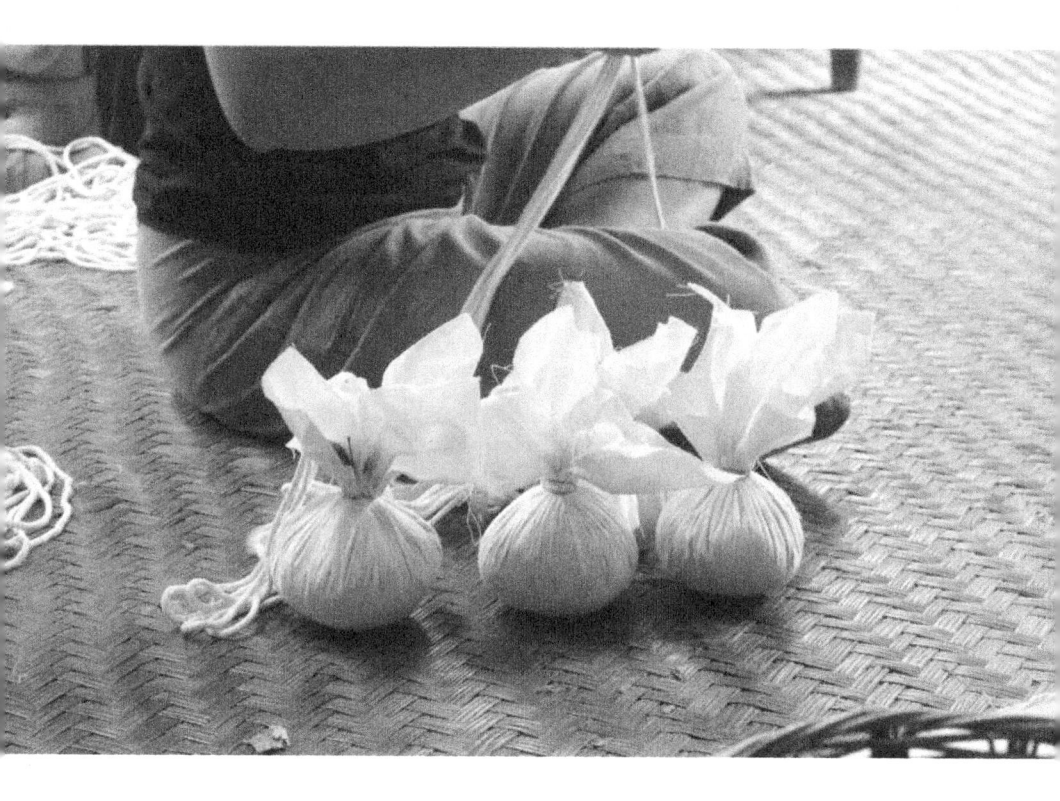

8.Making herbal balls in Thailand, with white cotton fabric.

Most therapists use cotton. Cotton is soft and inexpensive, at least compared to linen and silk.

Bear in mind that natural fibers will be stained by plants that possess certain pigments (like eucalyptus and turmeric). These stains are NOT dirt, they are natural dyes. Thus, should you want to reuse your fabrics after washing them, these stains are not an issue. I do not consider them unsightly. However, if you believe that these dyes will be unappealing for some clients, do replace your fabric after each treatment.

In the spirit of recycling and upcycling, I never throw away the fabric I use in my herbal ball treatments, as long as it is intact. I discard (I compost it actually) the plant material always after one treatment. Then, I wash the fabric with hot water and soap in hand (if you put it in the washing machine with other clothes, they may be stained by the plant pigments), and let it dry. Then, the fabric will be sterilized when placed in steam.

Strings

The string you will use to tie your compress, should also be made from natural fibers. These can be cotton, hemp, yucca or another natural material. Smoother strings are more preferable, especially if you have to make a large quantity of herbal balls daily, as they will be softer for your hands. Rough strings may in fact hurt your hands, but this will never be an issue if you are making just 2-3 herbal balls daily.

In Thailand, most therapists use a white thread to tie the herbal compress. The white color creates a uniform and "clean" look. However, you could use a thread with a different color, like the one made from yucca fibers. The brown color will create an interesting contrast and a more "natural" look. Of course, this is a purely visual matter.

I have also seen some therapists who prefer to tie the herbal ball with a piece of fabric, which is cut from the same fabric that was used for the herbal ball. This is also an acceptable solution, although I have never done it.

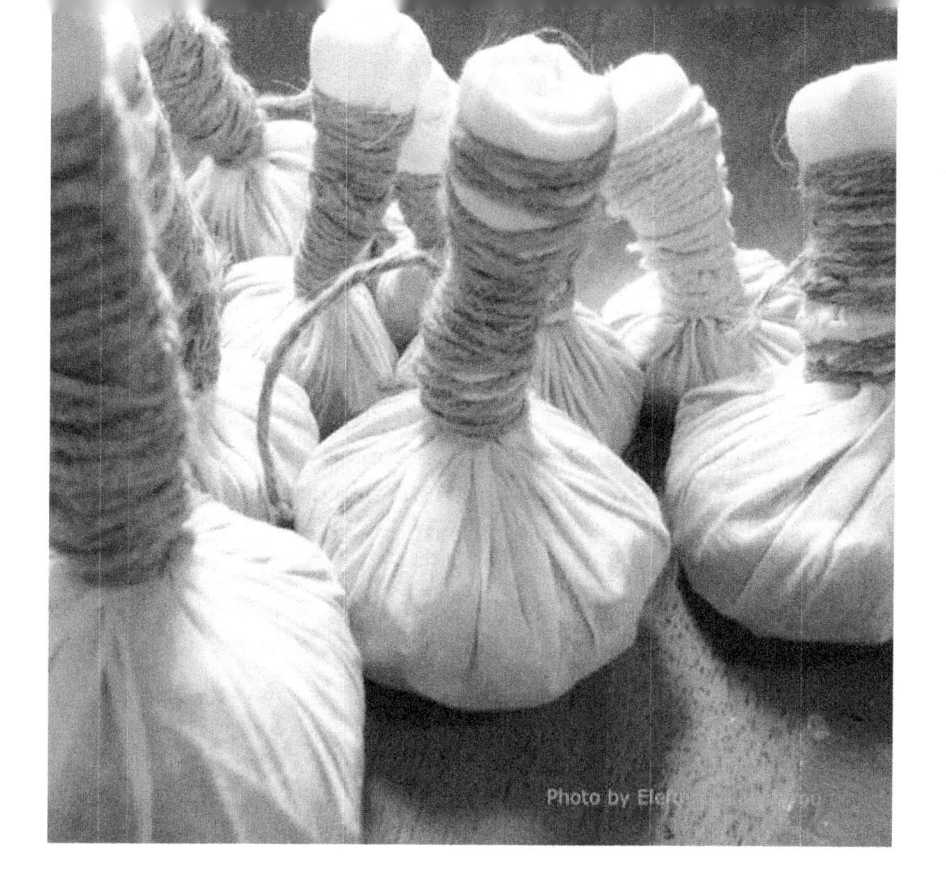

9. Herbal balls made in my school, during a Thai massage course. They are tied with yucca strings (except one in the back, which is tied with a white cotton string). Made with the "Rose Bud" method.

The important thing is to use an undyed string, which will not bleed after being exposed to the steam. Have fun exploring the options!

Luk Pra Kob and Yam Khang

When I was in Chiang Mai, Thailand, I had the chance to attend a class on Fire Foot Massage – or *Yam Khang*, as it is called in Northern Thailand. This traditional Lanna treatment involves fire (yes, real fire!), sesame oil, *phlai* water, a plough heated on charcoals, and of course foot massage.

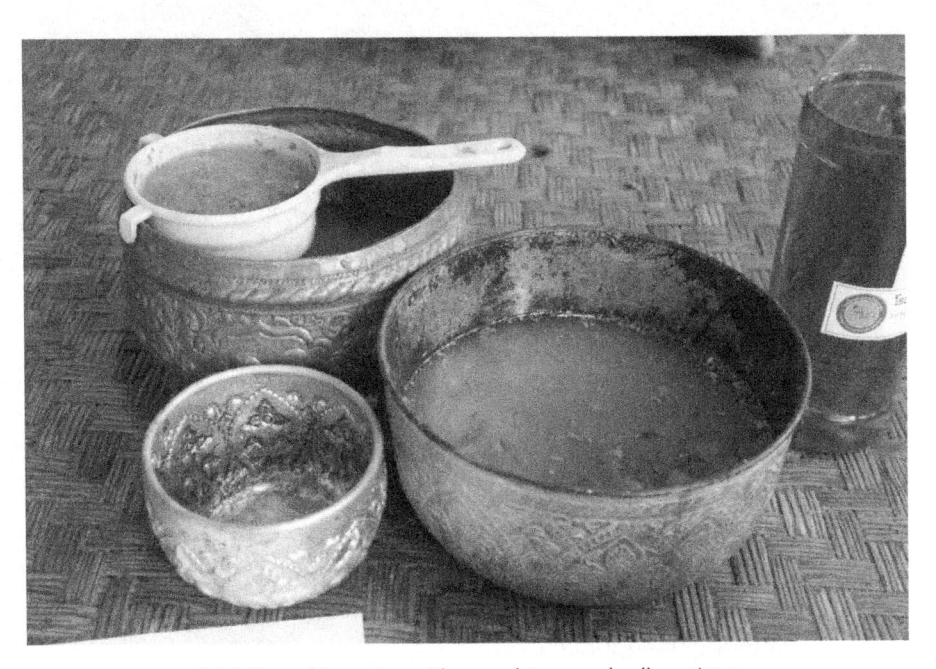

10. Making phlai water with a sandstone and yellow ginger.

The *Yam Khang* tools can also be used for herbal ball treatments. Before the treatment, the therapist prepares the phlai water by grinding phlai root with a sandstone (this is the Lanna, traditional method – you can use a modern grater).

Then, the grated phlai is mixed with water, and filtered. The therapist also uses sesame oil, in which he dips his foot in order to massage the receiver.

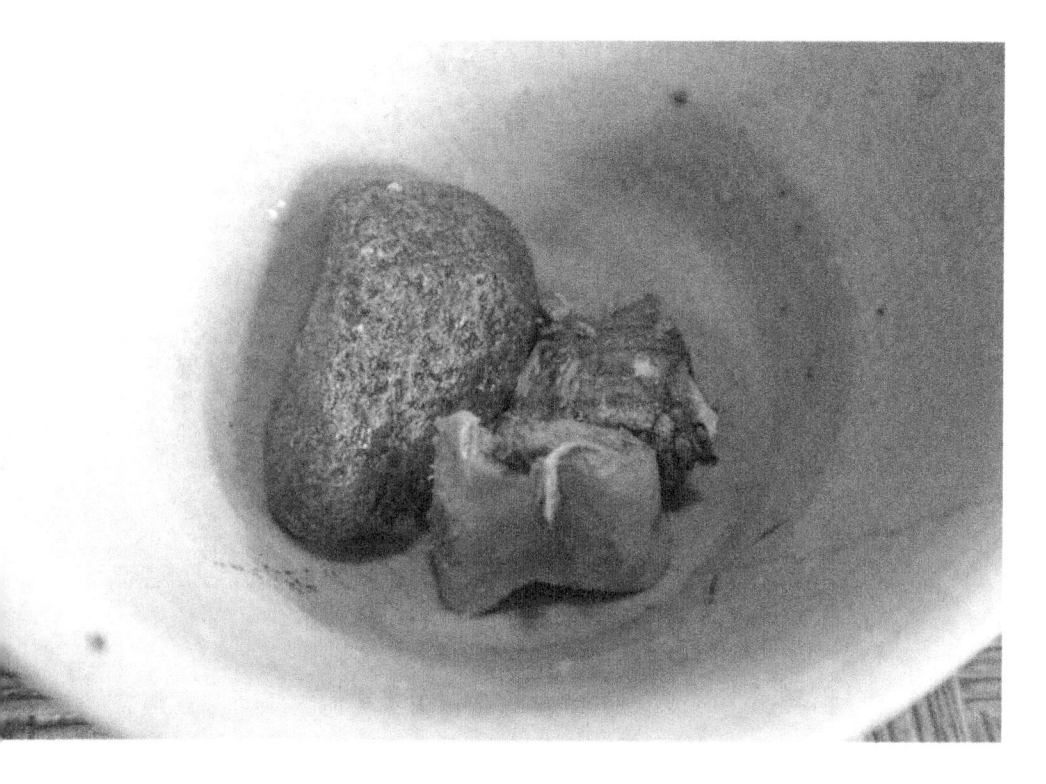

11. Sandstone and phlai ginger.

This is the process: The therapist dips his foot in the phlai water bowl and massages the receiver with his feet. After five dips in the phlai water, he dips his foot in the sesame oil bowl, and then touches his foot briefly on the hot plough. At this moment, fire emerges (it is pretty spectacular), which is supposed to warm and purify the therapist's foot. Then, the therapist massages the receiver with his foot.

Of course, there is no fire involved in the application of herbal balls, otherwise the herbs would be burned! The therapist dips the herbal ball in the phlai water bowl, and then rubs it on the hot plough at a brisk pace, 4-5 times – just so that it is heated.

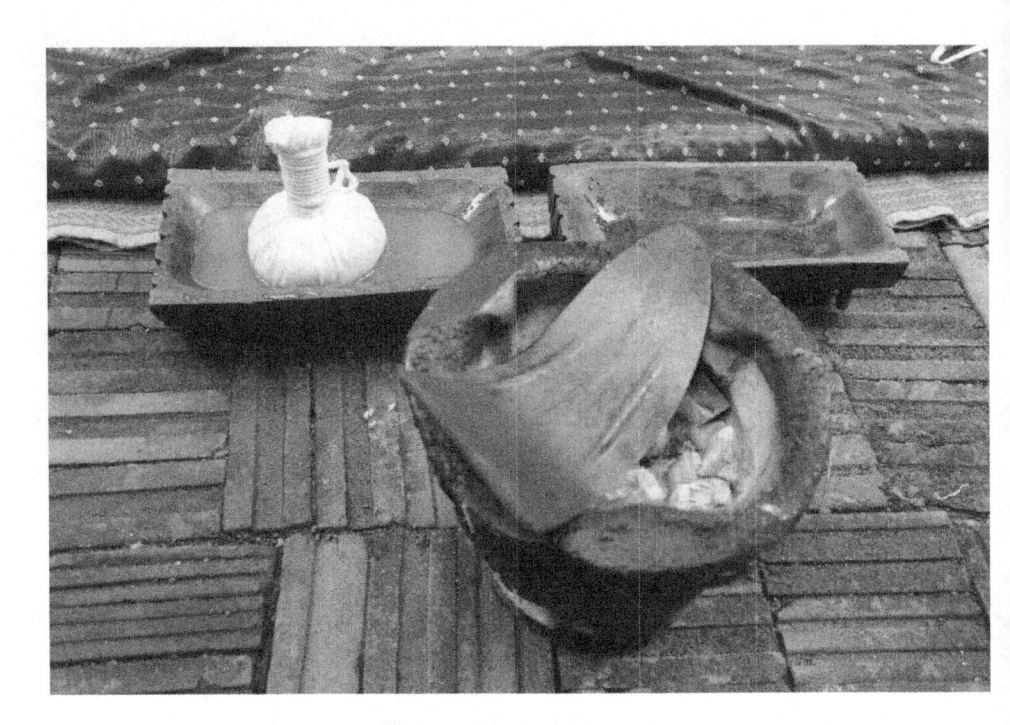

12. Plough heated in charcoals, for a more "primitive" (and sooo beautiful) application of herbal ball therapy, with the Yam Khang tools. You can see the herbal ball, dipped in phlai water. The other wooden bowl contains sesame oil.

Thus, in this method, the therapist uses his feet in order to massage the receiver, and includes the herbal ball in the treatment, by placing it wherever it is needed. When the herbal ball is no longer warm, the therapist rubs it again on the hot plough, and proceeds. Sesame oil is used in order to lubricate the receiver's body.

I have seen Thai therapists using a stick for support, in this treatment. Typically, this stick is inscribed with mantras that enhance protection and healing.

13. A stick bearing healing mantras, in Hang Dong Thai massage school in Chiang Mai, Thailand. It is used in their Luk Pra Kob treatments.

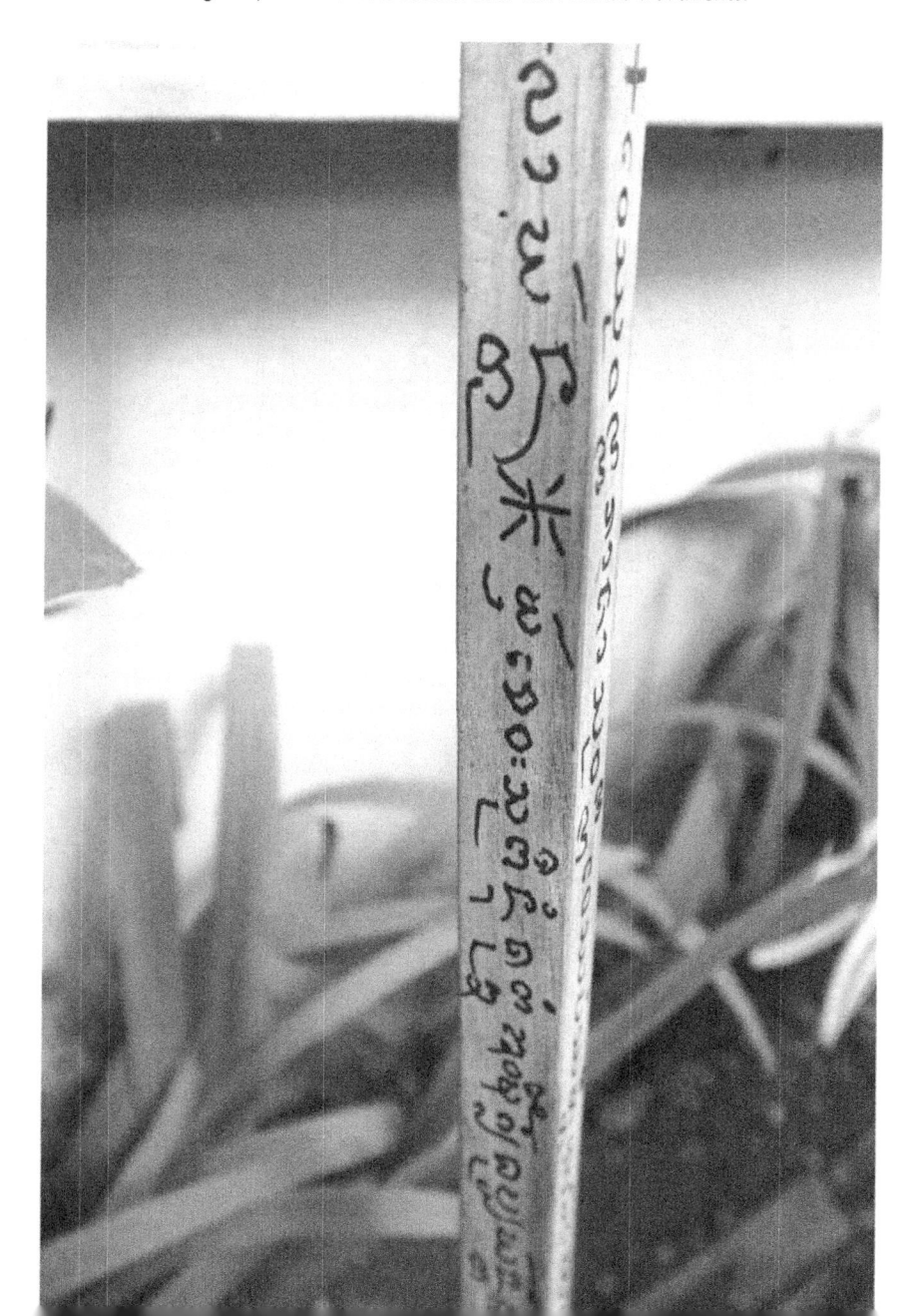

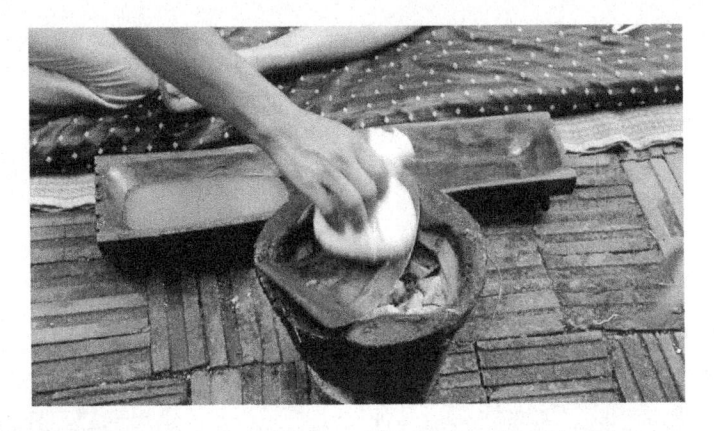

14. The therapist rubs the herbal ball on the hot plough in order to warm it.

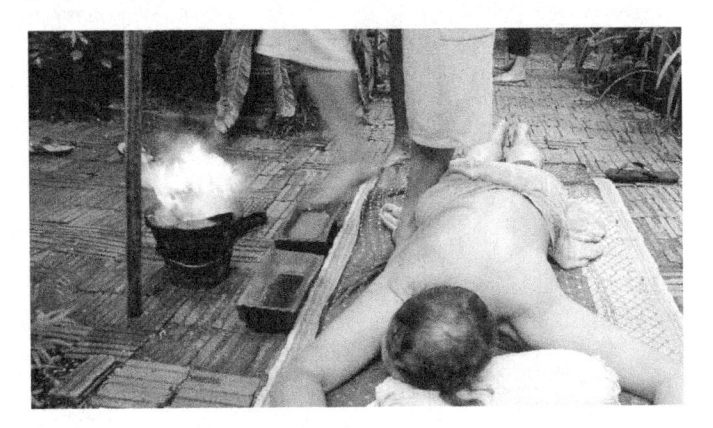

15. ...and a bit of Yam Khang – Fire Foot Massage – I wanted you to see a photo of this! You can see that the therapist is using the mantra-inscribed stick for support.

Obviously, this is very difficult (or impossible) to be done in the West. I wanted to include this traditional modality, because it was a part of my training in herbal balls in Thailand. I urge the reader to view this as an anthropologist would do.

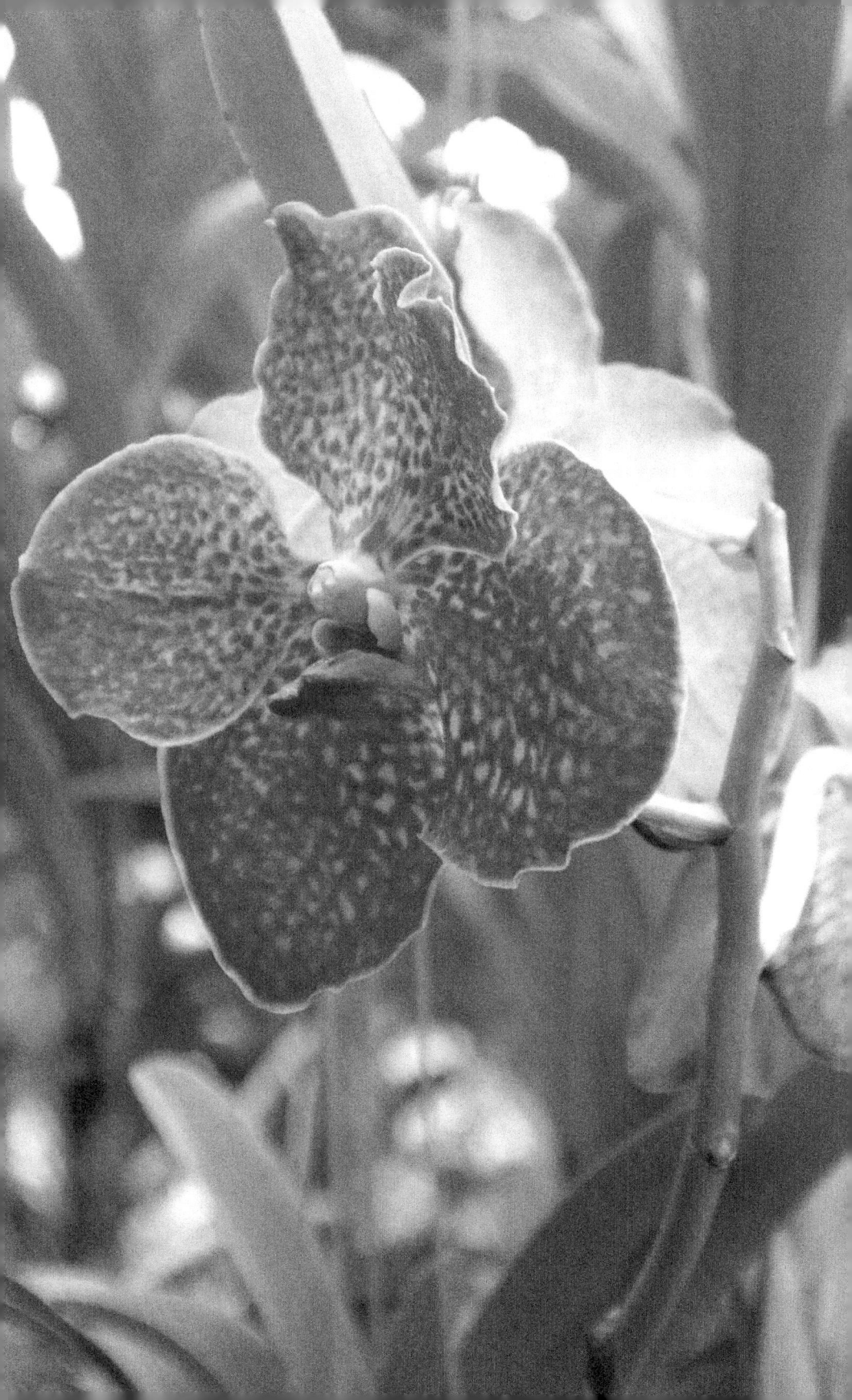

The Thai herbs

My original training was with Thai herbs. Many of them are readily available in herb stores in Europe and in the US, others can be foraged, while some will be unavailable in the West. Most of them can be obtained easily.

In my training in Thailand, most of the herbs were fresh. It is possible to mix fresh and dried herbs. Bear in mind that while packs that contain dried herbs can be stored indefinitely, the fresh herbs will deteriorate quickly. Of course, the commercial balls which are sold in stores contain exclusively dried herbs.

In order to make a basic herbal compress for musculoskeletal problems and respiratory disorders, you can make a mix containing the following herbs. I will suggest some detailed recipes in another section of this book. For the moment, let's begin by examining the herbs and their properties.

Eucalyptus

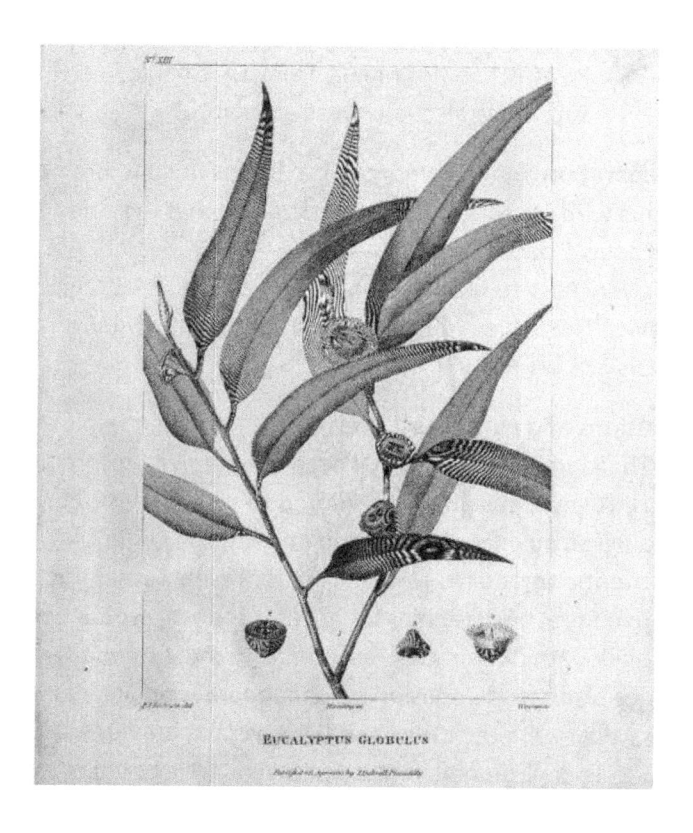

Latin name: Eucalyptus globulus (other Eucalyptus species can also be used).
Part used: leaves

Indications:

- Antipyretic. It can be used in the acute phase of the common cold.
- Muscle relaxant. A very useful herb for any type of muscle aches.
- Excellent for treating sinusitis.

- Suitable for the common cold and cough (strong expectorant).
- It is beneficial for oily skin and acne.
- Its effect comes mainly from 1,8 cineole, a substance also known as eucalyptol.

Preparation: In the compress, the leaves are cut into strips with scissors. It is best when fresh, but the dried herb has a decent effect as well.
It is very easy to identify, forage, dry and store eucalyptus leaves. The leaves will dye your fabric permanently, if its fibers are natural.

Cautions and concerns: Eucalyptus is not an endemic tree of Thailand. It has somehow become invasive. According to H. Zegeye, it is often considered to have undesirable ecological qualities such as depletion of soil water and nutrients, aggressive competition for resources with native flora, unsuitability for erosion control, production of allelopathic chemicals that suppress the growth of other plants and provision of inadequate food and habitat for wildlife. On the other hand, Eucalyptus provides multiple environmental and socio-economic benefits. It is useful for provision of wood and other products thereby reducing the pressure on the natural forests, conservation of soil and water, rehabilitation of degraded lands, fostering the regeneration of native woody species, provision of food and habitat for wildlife, drainage of swampy areas, mitigation of climate change and provision of amenity[ix].

Thus, therapists continue to use the herb in Thailand, although I have seen some who prefer not to add it in their mixes.

Phlai ginger

ZINGIBER CASSUMUNAR.—Roxb.—Miq

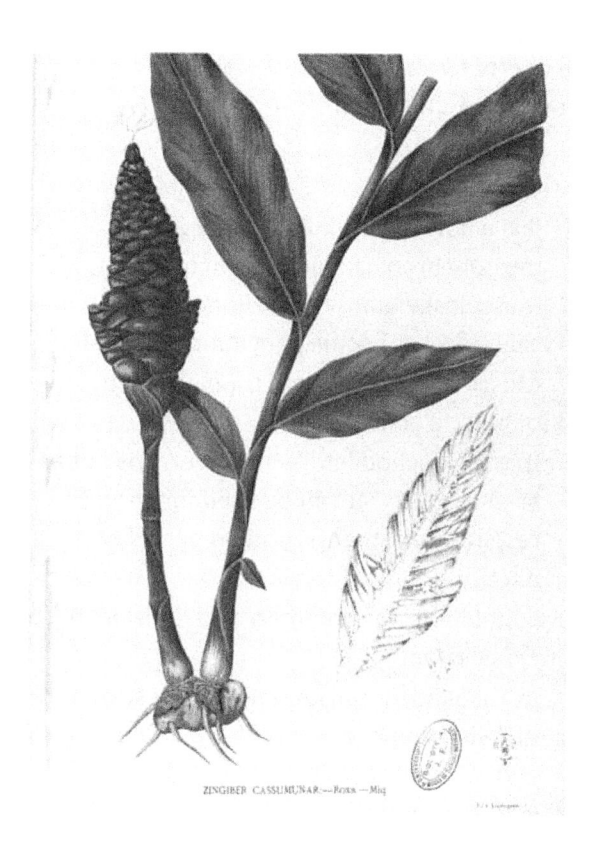

Latin name: Zingiber cassumunar
Part used: root (preferably fresh)

Indications:
Its Thai name is Phlai, and you may hear some Thais calling it "yellow ginger" in English. It is a potent bronchodilator, anti-inflammatory and antitussive herb.

It is frequently added in the compresses. I have also observed some traditional Thai therapists grinding it and mixing it with water. This "phlai water" is then used in Yam Khang (a traditional Lanna treatment involving fire) and an alternative application of hot herbal massage. More on this exciting stuff later!

- It is a potent anti-inflammatory herb. Add it in any mix for chronic inflammation of the musculoskeletal system. Bonus: it has none of the side effects of some conventional NSAIDs.
- Muscle relaxant. A very useful herb for any type of muscle aches.
- It is a bronchodilator – however, it is not as strong as eucalyptus. It can be used for chronic respiratory ailments, both in herbal packs, and as a tea.
- Suitable for the common cold and cough (strong expectorant).
- In Thailand, it is also used for digestive disorders of "wind" type (a term that could be associated with ailments like irritable bowel syndrome, or with symptoms like abdominal distention). I was told that phlai is considered a "cooling" herb, in contrast with common ginger (Zingiber officinale), which Thais consider "hot".

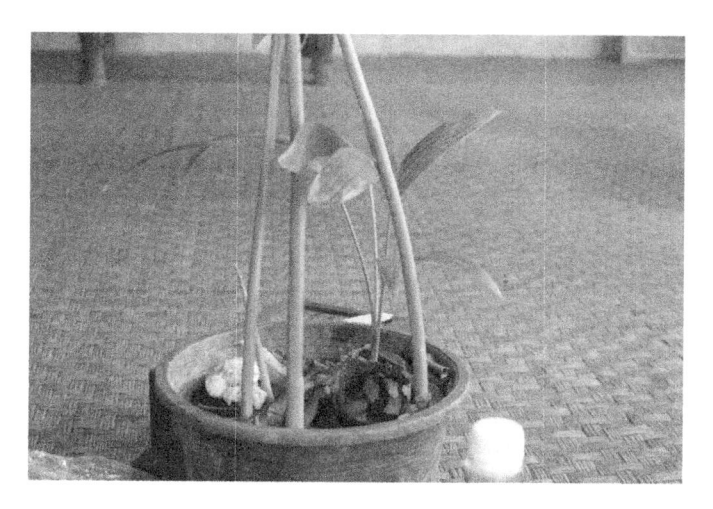

16. Phlai growing in a pot, in Chiang Mai. It is very easy to grow this plant. If protected from snow and extreme cold weather, it can be cultivated in temperate climates as well. Photo courtesy of Elefteria Mantzorou.

Preparation: Cut the rhizome in thin slices, and add it in the mix. There is no need to peel it.

Cautions and concerns: It leaves a slight yellow stain on hands, which is washed off easily (it may remain for half an hour or so).

It is hard to find this herb in the West (at least in Greece, where I am based). I have found it only frozen in shops that sell items for Thai cuisine, and it was expensive. I have not been able to find it in powdered form. Hence, I substitute it with common ginger in my herbal balls.

Camphor

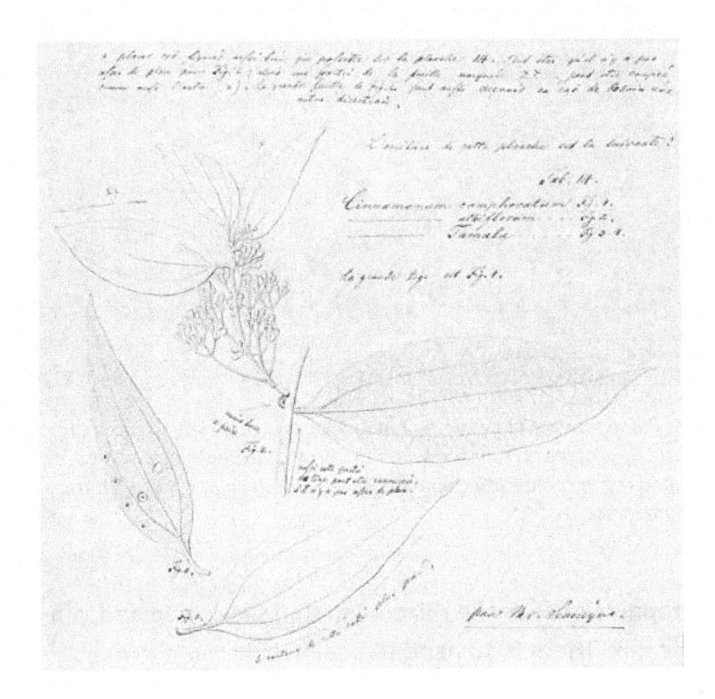

Latin name: Cinnamomum camphora

Part used: Resin. It is derived from the wood, and it is sold as a powder or in tablets.

Indications:

- It can increase the blood flow locally.
- Muscle relaxant and anti-inflammatory. A very useful herb for any type of muscle aches and any type of inflammation in the musculoskeletal system. Its effectiveness increases when used with peppermint.
- Suitable for the common cold – use it during the acute phase.

- Camphor is an important antitussive herb, and it can be used for any respiratory disorder.
- Its effect comes mainly from the ketone camphor (yep, it has the same name with the herb).
- It is believed that it purifies the meridians and the energy body.
- It is used in herbal inhalers for respiratory ailments (e.g. in the famous Thai *ya dom* inhalers).

Preparation: Camphor is usually sold in tablets. It should be pulverized in a mortar. Use up to 1 tablet of camphor per session. That's about 1 1/5 teaspoonful.

Cautions and concerns: Camphor should not be used in epileptic patients or during pregnancy and breastfeeding (because of the ketones it contains). It is unsuitable for kids. Do not exceed dosage. NEVER take camphor orally.

Fun Fact

The camphor tree belongs to the Lauraceae botanical family, which is quite ancient.

The family was widely distributed on the Gondwana supercontinent (600 to 530 Ma, that is million years ago). The continents' shape then, was very different from today. So, some trees of this family (and of many other botanical families as well) grew where there is sea now.

Kaffir lime

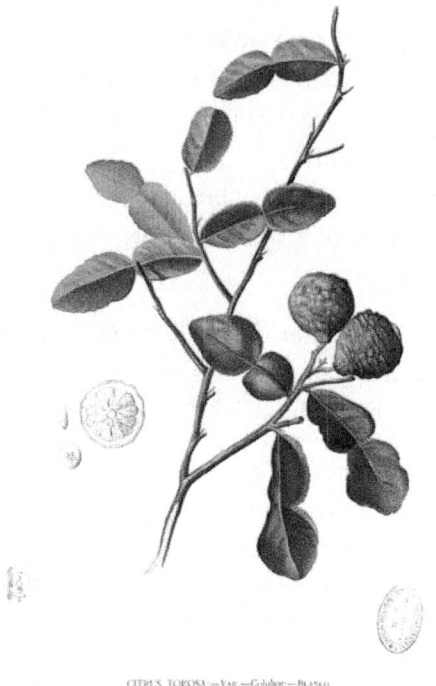

Latin name: Citrus hystix
Part used: rind (sometimes the leaf is also used).

Indications:

- While Thai cuisine – and other Southeast Asian cuisines – use only the leaf of this plant, the Thai therapists use mostly the rind.
- It slightly warms the muscles. It is added in the recipe for rheumatic, muscle and joint pain.
- Its euphoric fragrance is helpful for mental relaxation.

Preparation: Cut the fresh leaves in stripes with scissors. The rind should be cut in slices with a knife.

Cautions and concerns:
Do not exceed dosage, because it may be irritating for the skin. The Thai name of the plant is Makrut. If you cannot find kaffir lime, use the common lime instead. The most distinctive feature of this citrus is its bumpy exterior.

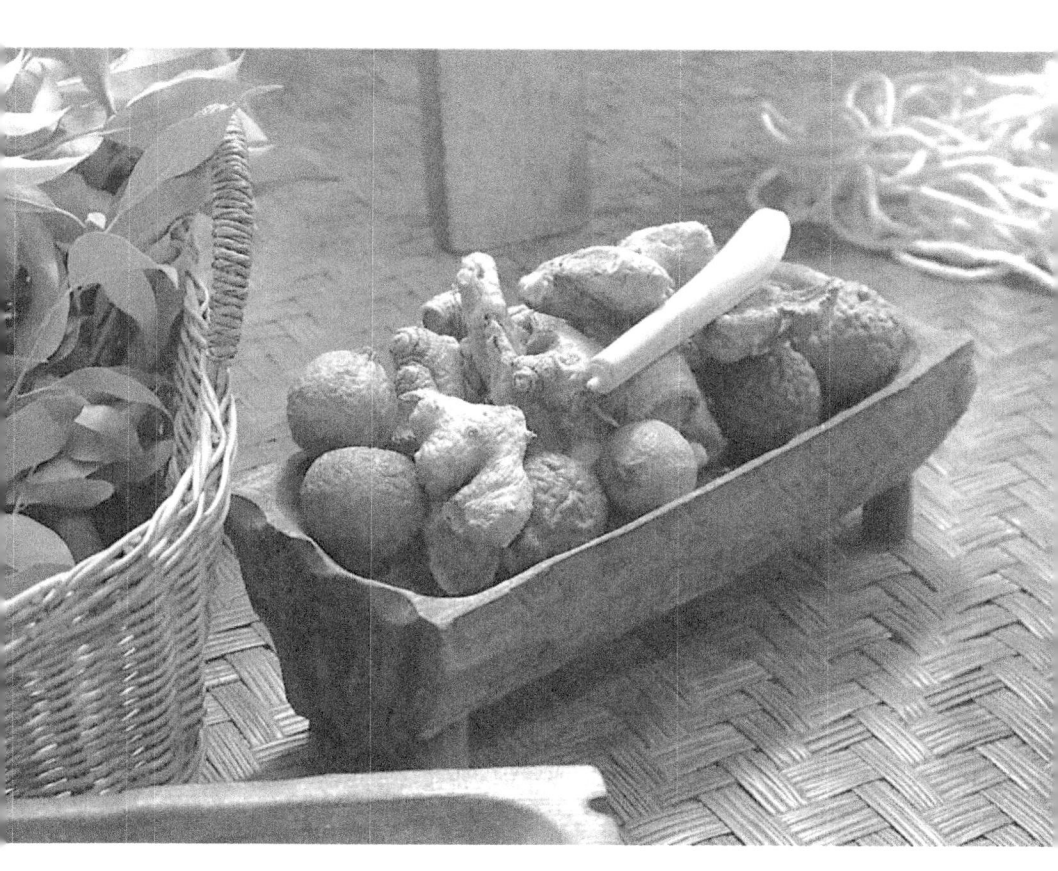

17. Kaffir lime, lemongrass and phlai, ready to be sliced and mixed in herbal balls. This photo was shot by Elefteria, in a massage school in Chiang Mai, Thailand.

Thai mint

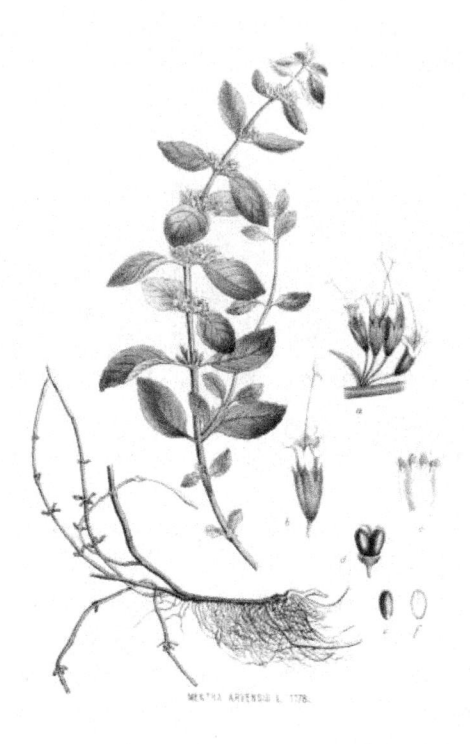

Latin name: Mentha arvensis
Part used: leaves

Indications:

- Mint leaf is added in the recipe because of its potent analgesic and anti-inflammatory properties. This is in important herb for headaches, and in fact any kind of ache that affects the muscles, the nerves (very useful for sciatica and lumbago) and the joints. It is also a must for any kind of rheumatic pain.
- Its scent can ease stress and refresh the mind and the senses.

- Suitable for the common cold – use it during the acute phase. It is an effective expectorant, especially when used fresh. In fact, it can be used for any respiratory problem, like congestion, catarrh, asthma, bronchitis and sinusitis.
- The active substance is menthol. It is has long been known that it enhances the skin permeation of camphor. Menthol's analgesic properties are mediated through a selective activation of κ-opioid receptors.[x] Menthol also blocks voltage-sensitive sodium channels, reducing neural activity that may stimulate muscles.

Preparation: Cut the leaves in slices with scissors. The fresh herb is more effective, but it is also acceptable to use dried leaves.

The leaves of other Mentha species are also suitable: M. piperita, M. spicata, M. haplocalyx (this species is known as "Bo He" in Chinese Herbal Medicine).

Cautions and concerns:

People with G6PD deficiency should consult their doctor before using any kind of mint.

Turmeric

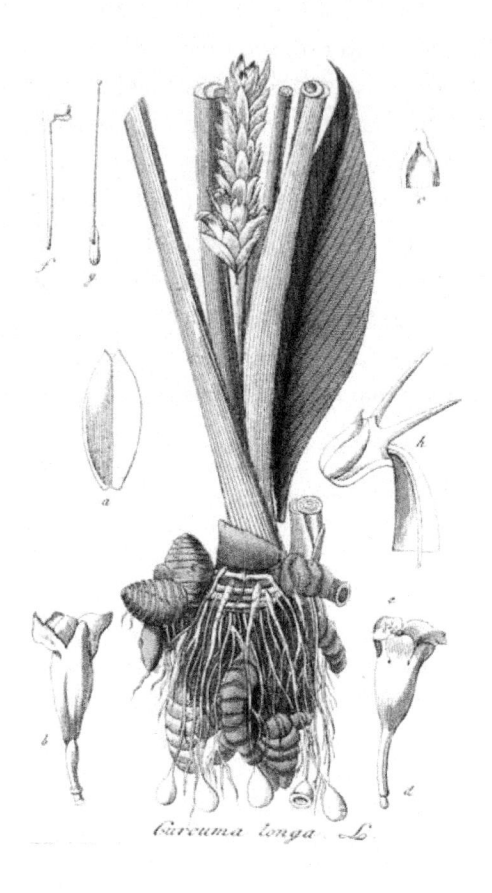

Latin name: Curcuma longa
Part used: root

Indications:

- Use turmeric root for any inflammation of the musculoskeletal system. It can be especially beneficial for osteoarthritis. Add it in any recipe for joint pain and compressed nerves.
- Turmeric may also help in the management of exercise-induced inflammation and muscle

soreness, thus enhancing recovery and subsequent performance in active people[xi].
- The active substance is curcumin, which has been under research for its anti-inflammatory effect.

Preparation: In Thailand therapists use the fresh root, which is cut into thin slices. Turmeric powder (comes from the dried root) is also acceptable.

Use up to 1 teaspoonful of powder for one treatment.

18. Curcuma long growing wild, in Doi Inthanon National Park in Northern Thailand. Photo is courtesy of Elefteria Mantzorou.

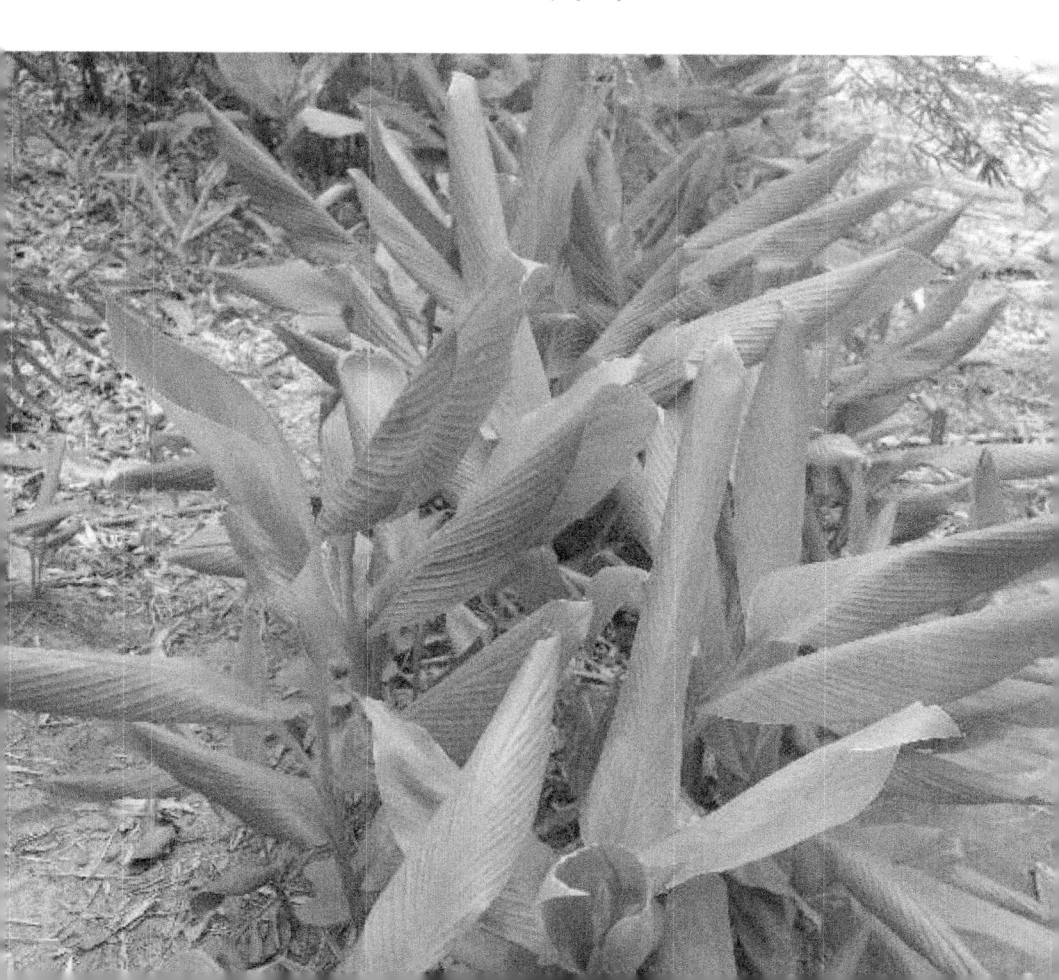

Cautions and concerns:

- Turmeric can stain the skin, clothing and other items. Be careful when you handle it. Its dye is pH-sensitive and will turn red if it comes in contact with alkaline substances, like washing soda.
- Sometimes, turmeric powder is adulterated with cheaper agents, like lead oxide and metanil yellow.

The Thai name for turmeric is khamin.

Lemongrass

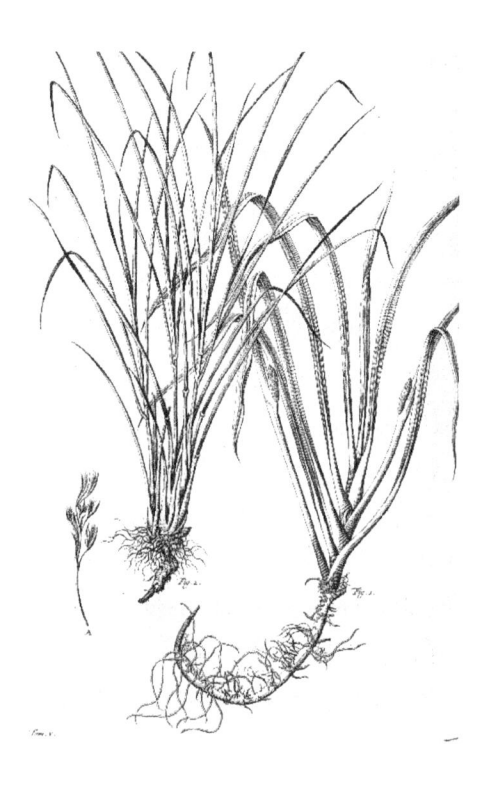

Latin name: Cymbopogon citratus
Part used: root and stem

Indications:

- The stem is added in the recipe mainly thanks to its elegant fragrance. It blends wonderfully with the aroma of camphor and eucalyptus.
- It has anxiolytic properties. This has been confirmed for the essential oil that is distilled from the leaves, and not for the whole herb. However, its aroma is still beneficial for stress.

- It is believed that it can "cool" the body, form an energetic point of view.

Preparation: It is best when used fresh. Just cut it in thin slices with a knife. Lemongrass looks like a small leek.

The dried herb is also acceptable. Just add a handful of it in the recipe. The Thai name of the herb is Ta khrai.

It is quite easy to grow lemongrass in your garden if you live in a warm temperate climate.

Cautions and concerns: None particular.

19. From top to bottom: Cinnamon leaf, lemongrass and tamarind leaf, on a piece of fabric, before it is made into an herbal ball.

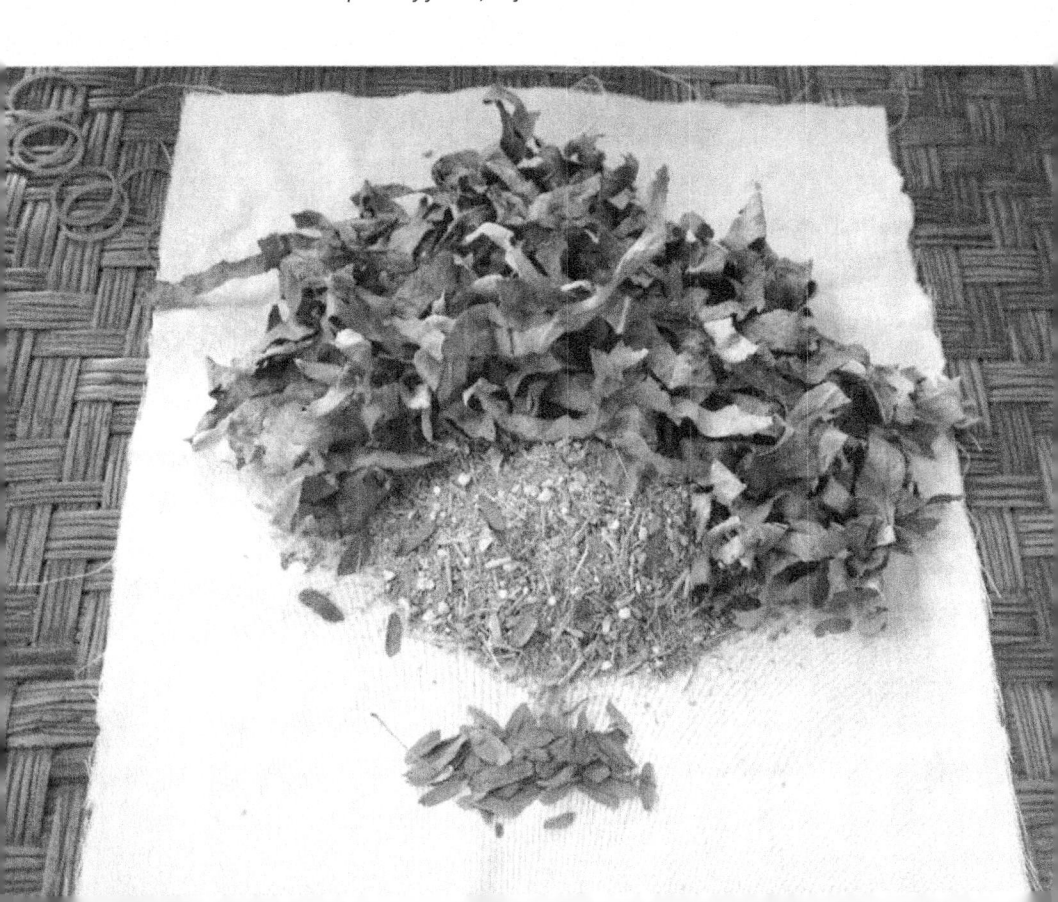

Tamarind

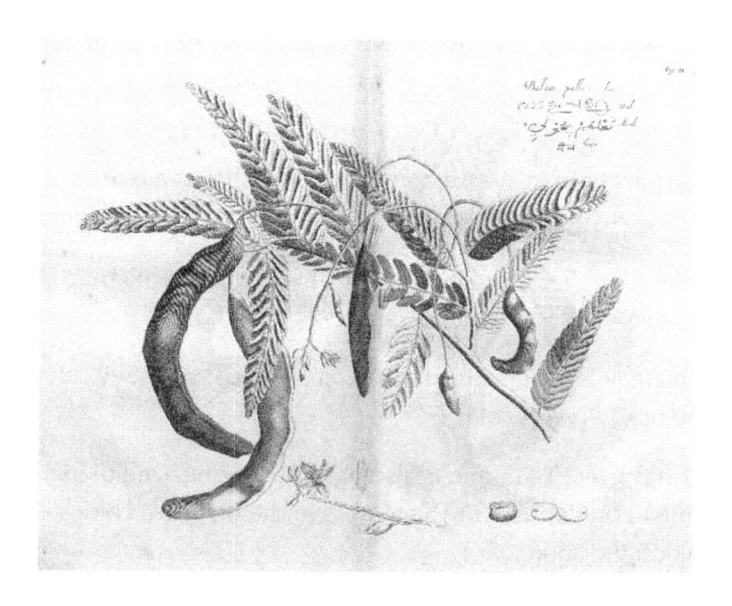

Latin name: Tamarindus indica
Part used: leaf and / or pulp

Indications:

- The pulp, which is extracted from the pod-like fruit, is added in the recipe mainly for its cosmetic properties.
- Tamarind pulp can moisten and exfoliate the skin. For this purpose, it works well combined with turmeric in the herbal pack.
- Since it possesses anti-inflammatory properties, the pulp can also be added in recipes for muscle and joint pain. It will always have the extra bonus of moistening the skin!
- Tamarind leaves can promote lactation, when added in the compress.

- Tamarind leaves also possess anti-inflammatory properties.
- Tamarind leaves have an analgesic effect, and thus are indicated for menstrual cramps.

Preparation: In Western countries, you have to buy tamarind pulp from stores that sell "ethnic" food supplies.

Use about 5 – 15 ml pulp for each session. Cut the pulp in small pieces with a knife.

The leaves should be cut in slices with scissors. They can be used dry as well.

Other uses: Tamarind is also used in cooking. One of its most popular uses in Thailand, is in the dish tom khlong – a hot and sour soup.

Cautions and concerns:

Some people can be allergic to tamarind. The possible symptoms of this allergy may include itching, hives and eczema. In spite of the fact that this pertains mostly to the ingestion of the herb, it could happen also with skin contact.

I have not been able to find tamarind leaves in the West, in any form. Thus, feel free to exclude the particular ingredient from your mixes.

Cumin

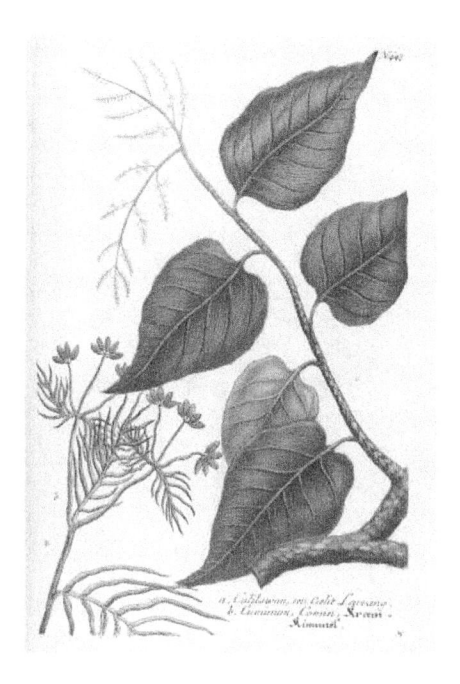

Latin name: Cuminum cyminum
Part used: seed

Indications:

- The seed is added in the recipe as an ancillary herb, mainly for its analgesic and muscle relaxant properties.
- Not suitable for cosmetic recipes.

Preparation: Use the whole or ground seed. Add up to one teaspoonful for each treatment.

Cautions and concerns: None particular. Do not exceed dosage, because it may be irritating for the skin.

Jasmine

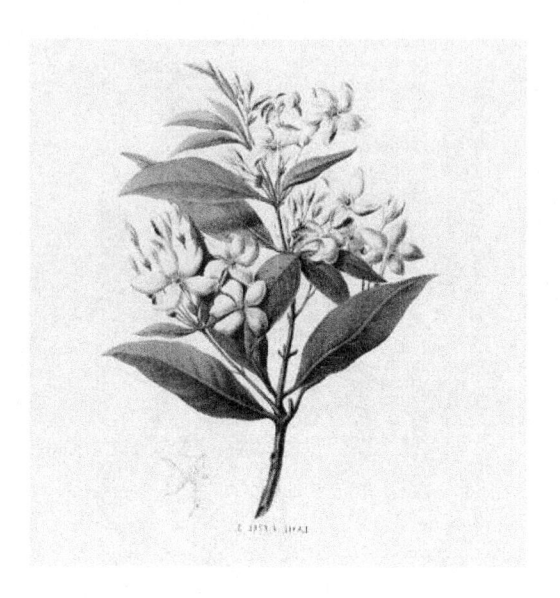

Latin name: Jasmin arabicum
Part used: flower

Indications:

- The jasmine flowers are added in the recipe mainly thanks to their fragrance, which has an anti-stress effect.
- As a secondary action, jasmine can be used in recipes for respiratory problems. Add it in mixes for chronic asthma, bronchitis and bronchospasm.

Preparation: It is best to use the fresh flowers. The dried flowers have almost no fragrance.

Cautions and concerns: None particular.

Thai herbs generally hard to find in the West

I will list some herbs that I saw they were being added in herbal packs recipes in Thailand, but are hard to find in Europe. Well, at least in Greece, where I live.

Occasionally, I have found some of these herbs (like Galangal) frozen, in ethnic food stores. Others (like cinnamon leaves or zerumbat ginger) were simply impossible to find.

Although nothing beats the unique aroma of the Thai herbal balls I had the luck to smell in Thailand, you can still make a decent herbal pack with the herbs I listed in the previous section. And it will still have a wonderful aroma, and a therapeutic effect. Yep, most of them can be successfully substituted.

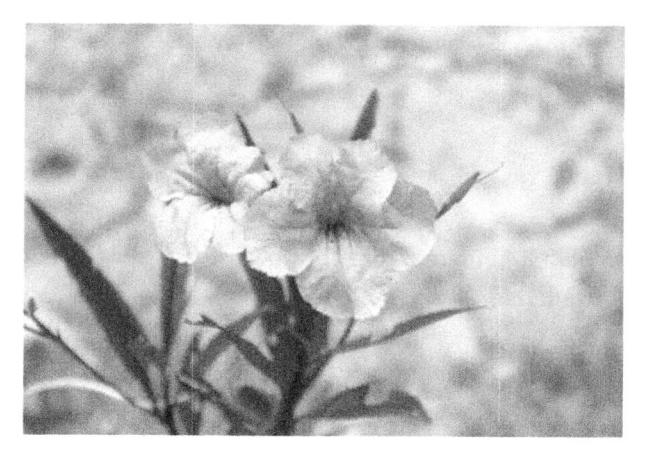

20. Ruellia tuberosa growing wild in a Karen hill tribe village, in Doi Inthanon National Park, Thailand. Its medicinal uses are currently under research, especially those pertaining to the treatment of diabetes [xii].

Cinnamon leaf

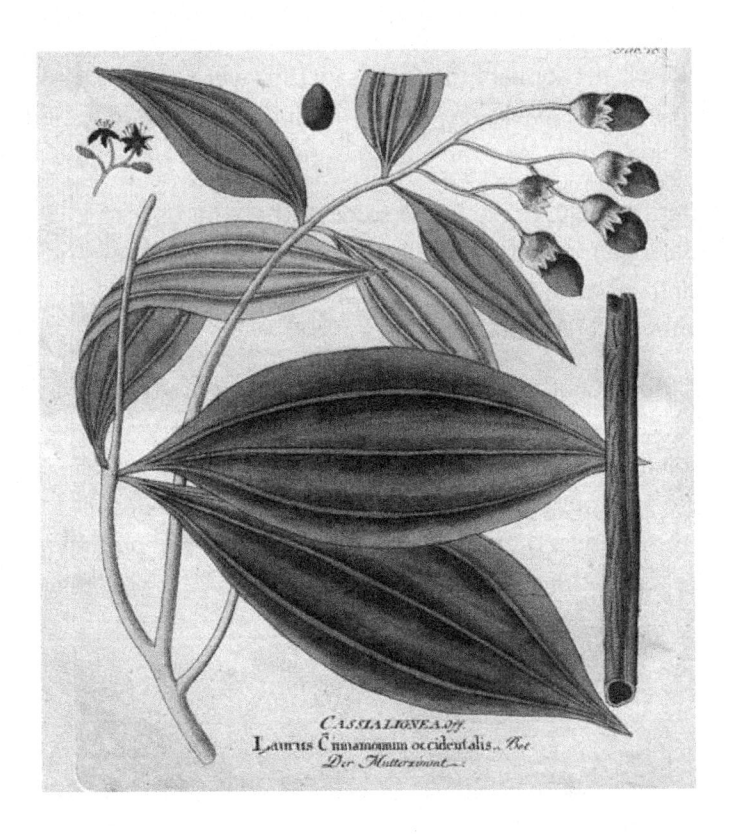

Latin name: Cinnamomum verum
Part used: leaf

Indications:

- Cinnamon leaf has a wonderful aroma, which has an anti-stress effect. The aroma of the leaf is more "medicinal" in comparison with that of the bark. This is because the bark derives its fragrance from the aromatic compound called cinnamaldehyde, which has a sweet aroma. Cinnamon leaf contains little cinnamaldehyde and

a high concentration of eugenol (hence the "medicinal" aroma).
- It warms the muscles. It is added in the recipe for rheumatic, muscle and joint pain.

Preparation: Cut the fresh leaves in stripes with scissors. Use about 1 spoonful for each herbal ball.

Cautions and concerns:
- Do not exceed dosage, because it may be irritating for the skin. Cinnamon leaf contains a high concentration of eugenol, a substance which can be caustic (this is a concern mostly for the essential oil).
- Although cinnamon bark can be purchased anywhere, this is not the case with the leaves.
- Never use cinnamon bark, because it can be irritating for the skin.

Alpinia galanga

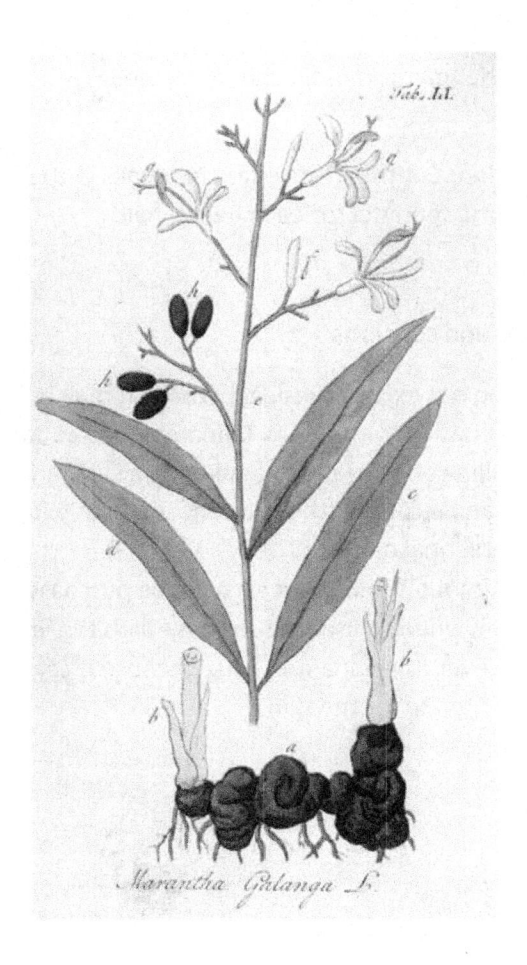

This is a very hot herb and spice, widely used in Thai cuisine. The Thai name is Khaa (internationally known as Siamese ginger, or Ginza). The root is frequently added in the compresses, although phlai ginger is more frequently used.

It is one of four plants known as galangal and is differentiated from the others with the common name lengkuas, greater galangal, or blue ginger. It is the galangal used most often in cookery. It is valued for its use in food and for traditional medicine and is regarded as being superior to ginger. The rhizome has a pungent smell.

The word galangal, or its variant galanga, can refer in common usage to the aromatic rhizome of any of four plant species in the Zingiberaceae (ginger) family, namely:

- Alpinia galanga, also called greater galangal, lengkuas or laos.
- Alpinia officinarum, or lesser galangal.
- Boesenbergia rotunda, also called Chinese ginger or fingerroot.
- Kaempferia galanga, also called kencur, black galangal or sand ginger.

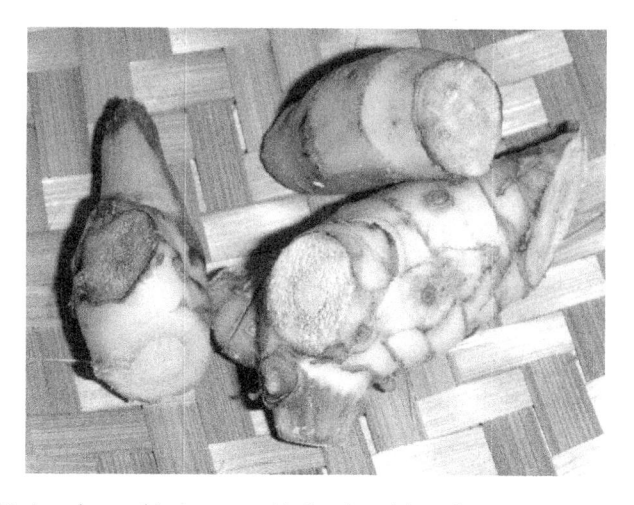

21. A. galanga rhizomes, cut. Notice the white color, in contrast with phlai, Cassumunar ginger, which has an intense yellow color.

While all varieties of galangal are closely related to common ginger, and all exhibit some resemblance to the hot, spicy flavor of ginger, each is unique in its own right, and galangals are not typically regarded as synonymous with ginger or each other in traditional Asian dishes [xiii], and in medicine.

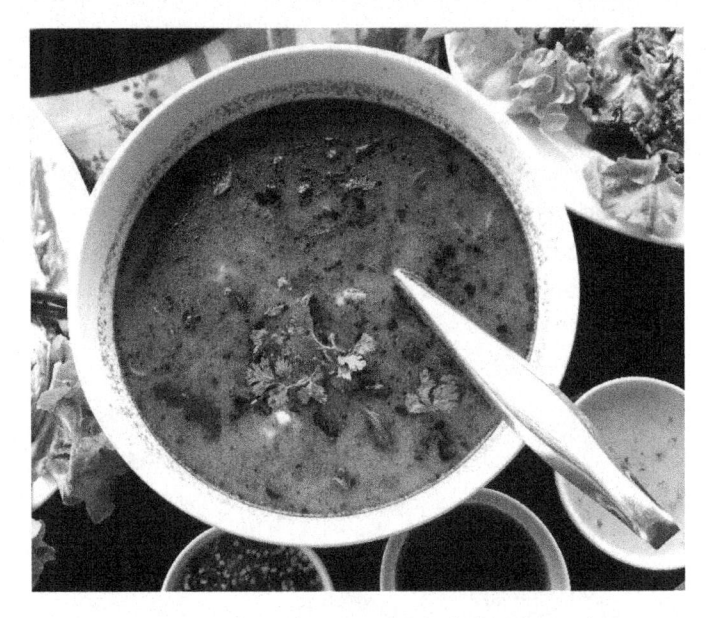

22. Tom yum soup. It is characterised by its distinct hot and sour flavours, with fragrant spices and herbs generously used in the broth.

Galangal is perhaps the most basic herb in the famous *tom yum* Thai soup. Depending on the quantity of galangal and chillies, it can be VERY hot!

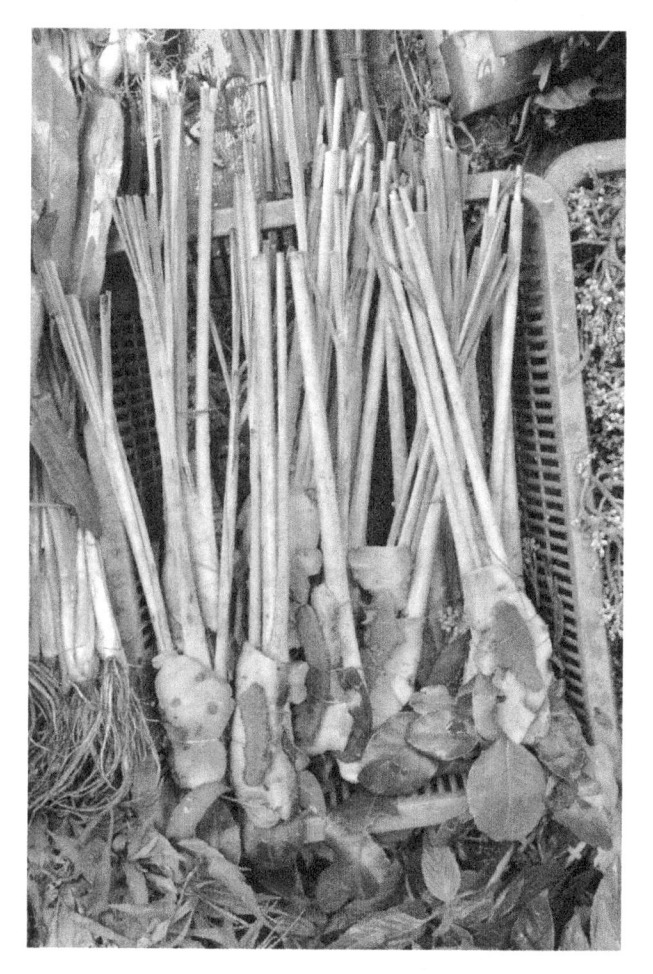

23. Ready-to-use for tom yum, bundles of lemon grass, galangal, lime leaves, and turmeric, are sold at Thai markets. [xiv]

Tom yum soup can be eaten during colds, as the herbs it contains are strong expectorants and diaphoretics. It includes fresh ingredients such as lemongrass, kaffir lime leaves, galangal, lime juice, and crushed red chili peppers. A paste from these ingredients is bottled or packaged and sold around the world.

I wanted to share with you some photos of Alpinia galangal I took in an Akha village, in Northern Thailand.

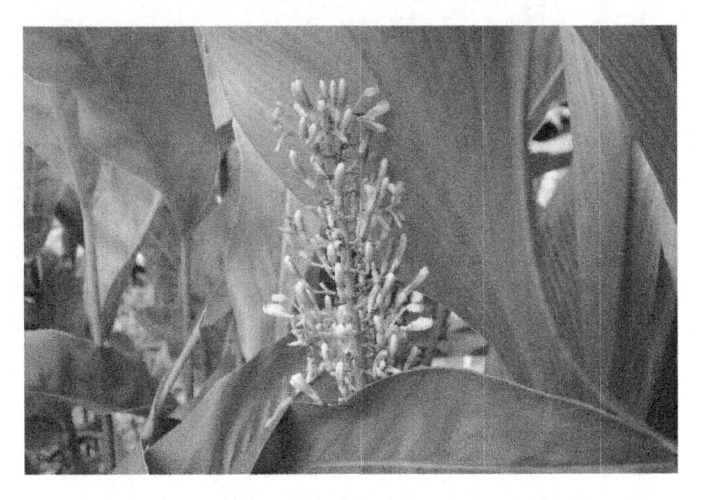

24. The beautiful galangal flower!

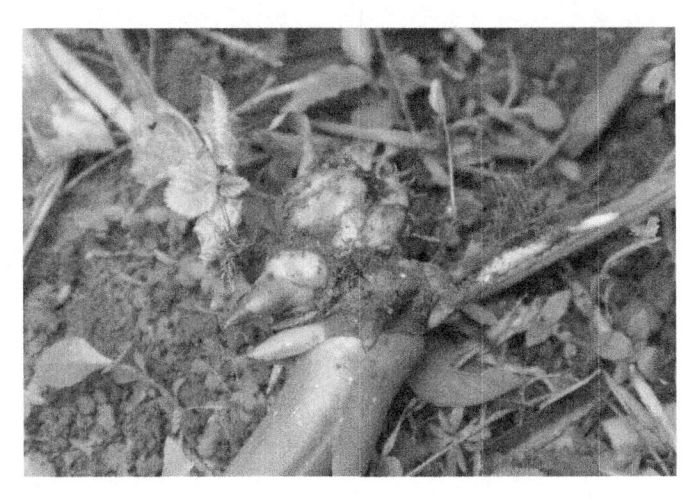

25. Galangal root. My Akha guide who found the plant, was ecstatic (I think he phoned his wife and told her to start preparing a soup!).

Zerumbet ginger (Zingiber zerumbet)

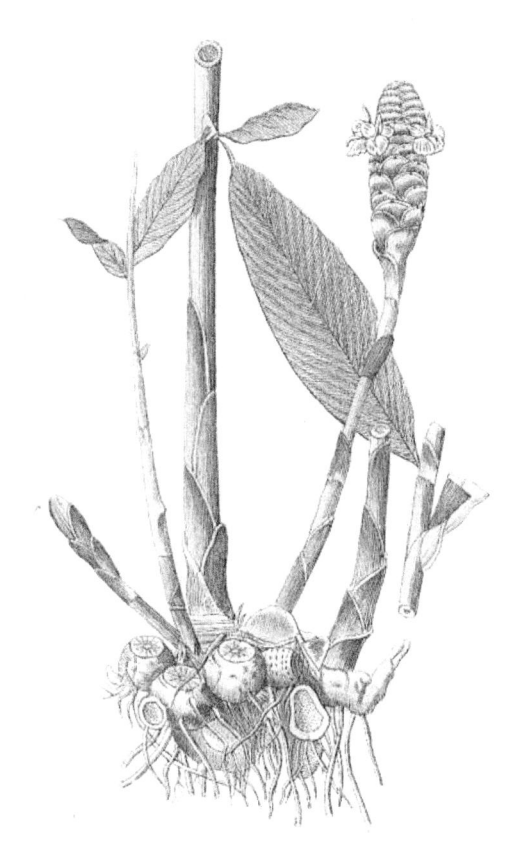

Amomum Zerumbet. L.

The Thai name of the herb is Ka Thue, and internationally it is known as Pinecone ginger. This is a potent herb. Very effective for tense muscles and injuries. The root is frequently added in the compresses.

This herb is also used in the indigenous medicine of Hawaii, for similar purposes.

Blumea balsamifera

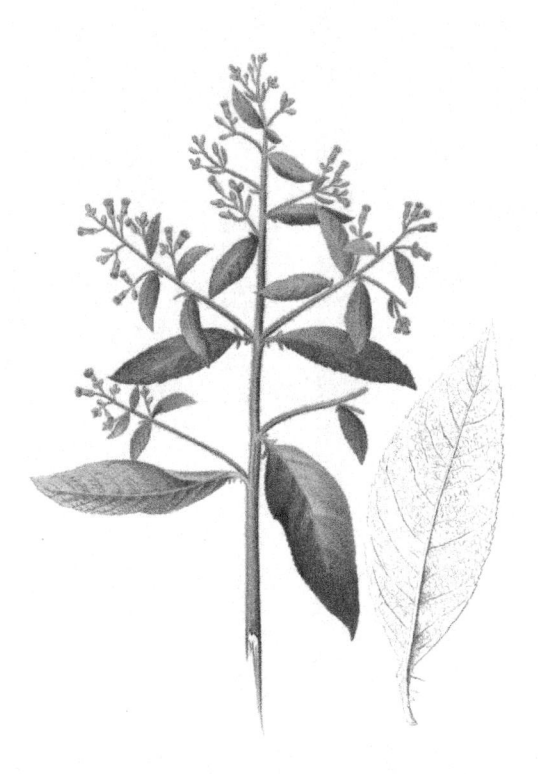

In Thai, this plant is called Naat. I have seen its leaves being added in the herbal steamer.

It is a strong expectorant, and it is also used for the treatment of infections. The leaf contains an essential oil, rich in camphor and limonene [xv].

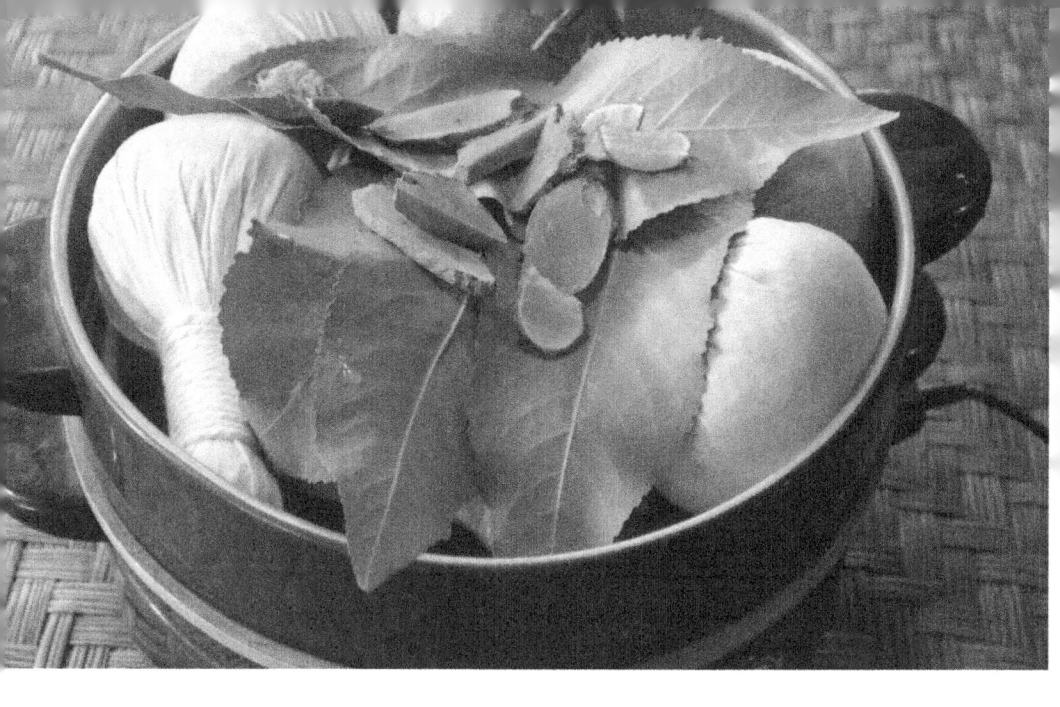

26. Naat leaves on top of herbal balls, along with phlai slices and kaffir lime. Ready for steaming!

Cardamoms

A Thai compress may also contain Cardamom leaves. These are the species used: Krawaan (Amomum krervanh), Reo krawaan (Amomum xanthioides) & Wan Sao Lowng (Amomum uliginosum).

These are also very hard to find in the West.

Other herbs

A Thai herbal compress may also contain Pandanus amaryllifolius (*bai toey hom* in Thai – added for its soothing aroma), and Piper longum (*dee-plee* in Thai).

Making herbal balls with Western herbs

Thai herbal ball therapy has such a good reputation for its anti-inflammatory and analgesic results, mainly thanks to the compounds contained in the medicinal plants of the Zingiberaceae botanical family. Now, the plants of this family have a pantropical distribution in the tropics of Africa, Asia, and the Americas, with their greatest diversity in Southeast Asia. Thus, as it was mentioned in the previous sections, some of them are not available in the West.

However, there are some Zingiberaceae plants that are readily available in the West, and at very affordable prices. Moreover, there are some Western herbs which also have a decent anti-inflammatory and analgesic properties.

Some of the Thai herbs that are added in recipes, are used mainly thanks to their aroma, which is an important factor in herbal ball treatments. The substitution of these herbs is of course, a much easier job in comparison to the substitution of the anti-inflammatory plants that contain compounds found in the Zingiberaceae botanical family.

So let's have a look at some herbs that are readily available in the West that can be added to herbal ball recipes.

Lemon

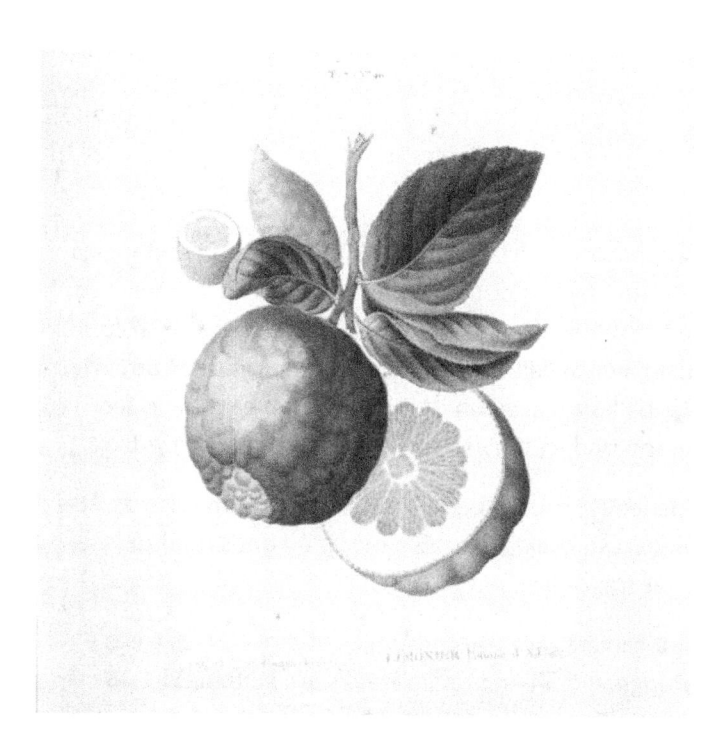

Latin name: Citrus limon
Part used: Leaf and rind

Indications:

- It is added in the recipe mainly thanks to its fragrance. The citrusy aroma somehow balances the "pharmaceutical" scent of the other herbs.
- The scent of the rind and the leaves has anxiolytic properties. Petitgrain, one of the most popular essential oils for stress and melancholy, is distilled from Citrus leaves.
- Suitable for the common cold – use it during the acute phase. The rind is considered an effective

expectorant (especially when consumed in an infusion, but it works well in poultices too).
- The rind and the leaves are also mild muscle relaxants (nowhere close to camphor or eucalyptus, but in any case they are cheap, and readily available, so why not use them as well?).

Preparation: Slice the rind in medium-sized rectangles (about 1 inch wide). If you are using fresh lemons, use only the rind and not the flesh, because the flesh contains juice, which will start dripping on the client's body when the ball is pressed on it! It is acceptable to use dried lemon rind, cut in very small pieces or pulverized.

The leaves should be cut in thin slices with scissors. Use only fresh leaves, because the dried ones tend to lose their fragrance.

You can actually use the leaves of most Citrus trees – orange and bitter orange leaves are suitable.

Cautions and concerns:
It is recommended to use organic lemons whenever possible, as the rind may have been heavily sprayed.

Have in mind that lemon rind contains pectin, a mucilaginous substance, which may make the herbal ball feel a bit "sticky" after heating. Of course, it is the white inner part of the citrus peel that is rich in pectin – if you use only the external rind, you will not have this "stickiness". By the way, pectin has demulcent properties, and it is great for your skin.

Ginger

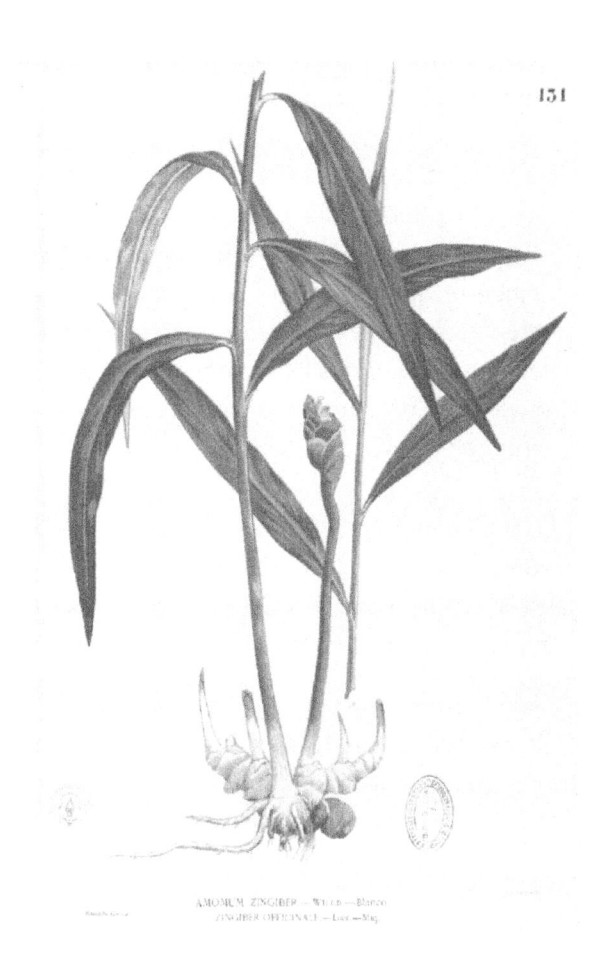

Latin name: Zingiber officinale

Part used: Root

Indications:

- It is a strong diaphoretic. It can be used in the acute phase of the common cold.
- Muscle relaxant and anti-inflammatory. A very useful herb for any type of muscle aches and any

type of inflammation in the musculoskeletal system.
- Suitable for the common cold and cough (strong expectorant, especially combined with eucalyptus leaf).
- It has a diaphoretic effect – that is, it can promote sweating during infections.
- Its effect comes mainly from the substance gingerol, and the volatile oils. However, the steaming of ginger transforms gingerol into zingerone, which is less pungent and has a spicy-sweet aroma. Zingerone is a particularly efficient free radical scavenger.

Preparation: It is best to use fresh ginger. It is very cheap and easily available. Cut it in small cubes with a sharp knife, and add it in the herbal ball mixture. You do not have to peel it.

Ginger powder is also easily available, but it is more expensive and, as I have found, not as effective as the fresh herb. However, you can use it.

Cautions and concerns: Always use ginger wrapped in cloth, otherwise it can be irritating for the skin.

The ginger family

Zingiberaceae or the ginger family, is a family of small to large herbaceous flowering plants, made up of about 50 genera. This family contains about 1600 known species of aromatic perennial herbs with creeping horizontal or tuberous rhizomes distributed throughout tropical Africa, Asia, and the Americas.

Many of the family's species are important ornamental, spice, or medicinal plants. Ornamental genera include the shell gingers (Alpinia), Siam or summer tulip (Curcuma alismatifolia), Globba, ginger lily (Hedychium), Kaempferia, torch-ginger Etlingera elatior, Renealmia, and ginger (Zingiber).

Spices include ginger (Zingiber), galangal or Thai ginger (Alpinia galanga and others), melegueta pepper (Aframomum melegueta), myoga (Zingiber mioga), korarima (Aframomum corrorima), turmeric (Curcuma), and cardamom (Amomum, Elettaria).

Some genera yield essential oils used in the perfume industry (Alpinia, Hedychium)[xvi].

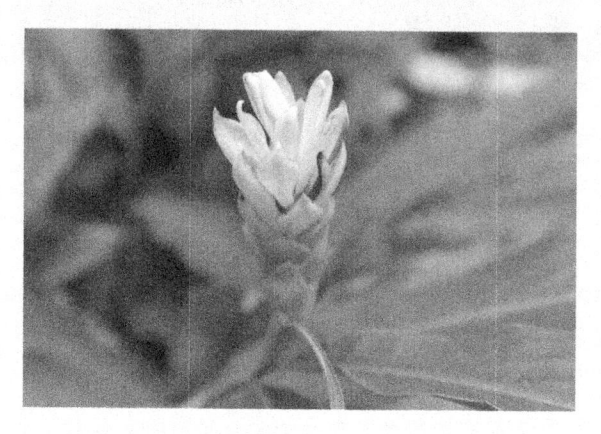

27. The beautiful flower of Alpinia purpurata.

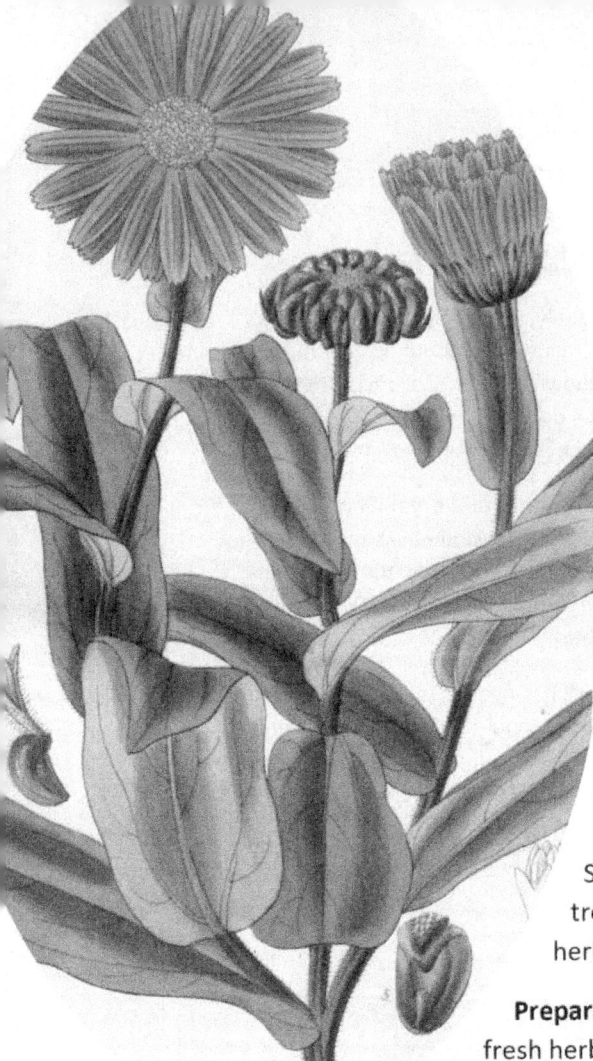

Calendula

Latin name: Calendula officinalis
Part used: leaf and flower

Indications:

Soothes the skin. Add it in recipes for people with inflamed, sensitive or damaged skin [xvii].

Suitable for cosmetic treatments that include hot herbal packs.

Preparation: It is best to use the fresh herb. Just cut it with a knife or scissors. The dried herb will also work.

Cautions and concerns: Will leave a yellow stain on fabric. Do not apply heat on burned skin. Do not use on people with allergies to Asteraceae family plants.

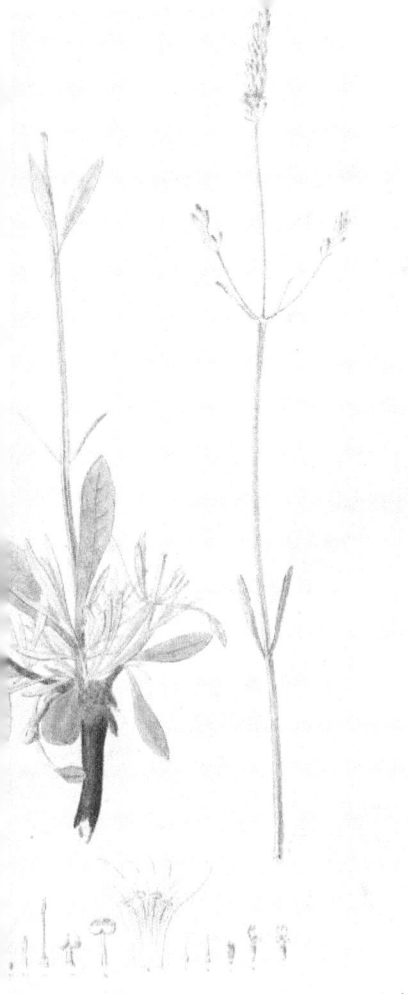

Lavender

Latin name: Lavandula officinalis
Part used: leaf, stem and flower.

Indications:

Soothes irritated and inflamed skin.

Suitable for acne.

Its aroma is indicated for stress and insomnia. Pairs well with chamomile and lemon balm for this.

Add it in recipes for chronic inflammation of the musculoskeletal system, as an ancillary herb.

Preparation: It is best to use the fresh herb. Just cut it with scissors. The dried herb will also work.

Cautions and concerns: None.

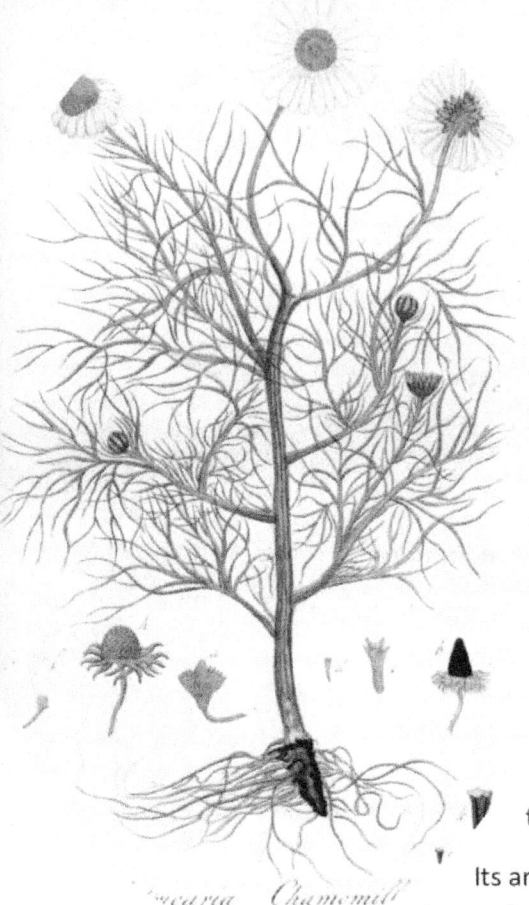

Chamomile

Latin name: Matricaria chamomilla

Part used: leaf, stem and flower.

Indications:

Soothes irritated and inflamed skin.

It can be used as an ancillary herb for chronic inflammatory conditions of the digestive system.

Its aroma is indicated for stress and insomnia. Pairs well with lavender and lemon balm for this.

Add it in recipes for chronic inflammation of the musculoskeletal system, as an ancillary herb.

Preparation: It is best to use the fresh herb. Just cut it with scissors. The dried herb will also work.

Cautions and concerns: Will leave a yellow stain on fabric. Do not apply extreme heat on sensitive skin. Do not use on people with allergies to Asteraceae family plants.

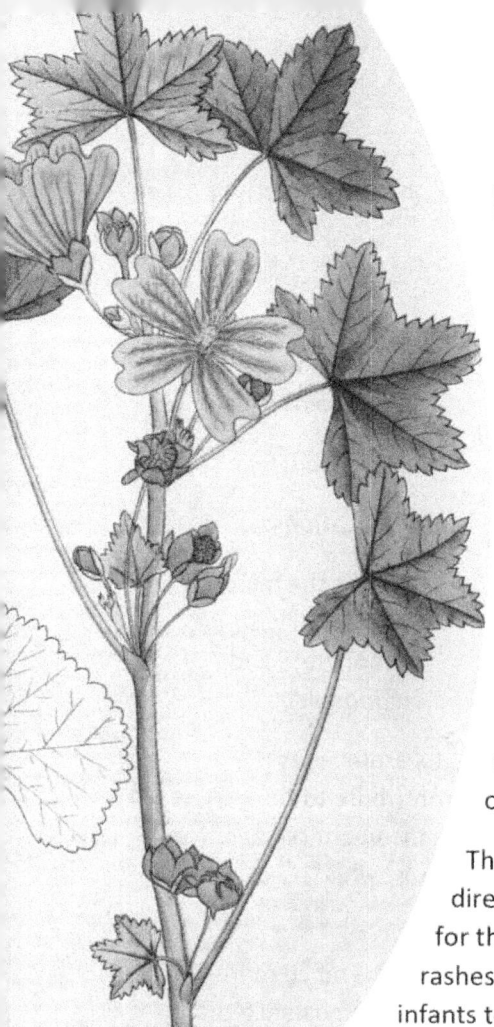

Mallow

Latin name: Malva sylvestris

Part used: leaf and flower. The flowers contain considerably more mucilage, which the main healing compound of this herb.

Indications:

Calms and nourishes the skin. A great herb for cosmetic herbal treatments.

The fresh herb can be applied directly on the skin as a poultice, for the treatment of wounds, rashes and boils. Suitable for infants too.

Preparation: It is best to use the fresh herb. Just cut it with scissors. The dried herb will also work.

Cautions and concerns: None. It is very easy to identify, forage and store this herb. Harvest responsibly.

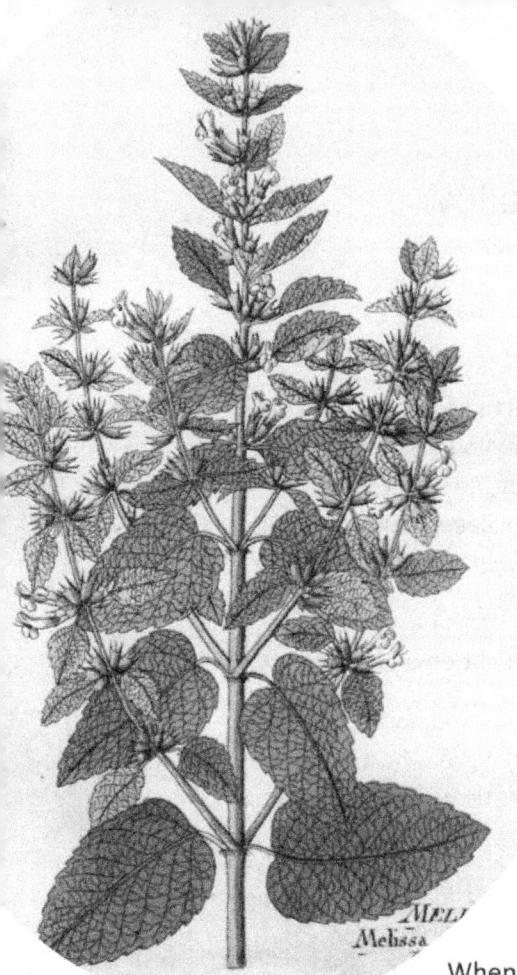

Lemon balm

Latin name: Melissa officinalis

Part used: leaf

Indications:

Calms the mind. Pairs well with lemongrass and chamomile.

Its aroma may contribute to the enhancement of cognitive functions, when used regularly.

When used fresh, it is much more fragrant. Thus, its aroma can balance the "pharmaceutical" scent of other plants.

Preparation: It is best to use the fresh herb – by the way, it is very easy to cultivate and propagate this plant, even at the balcony. Just cut it with scissors. The dried herb will also work.

Cautions and concerns: Use it with caution at people with hypothyroidism, although this applies mostly to the internal use of the herb.

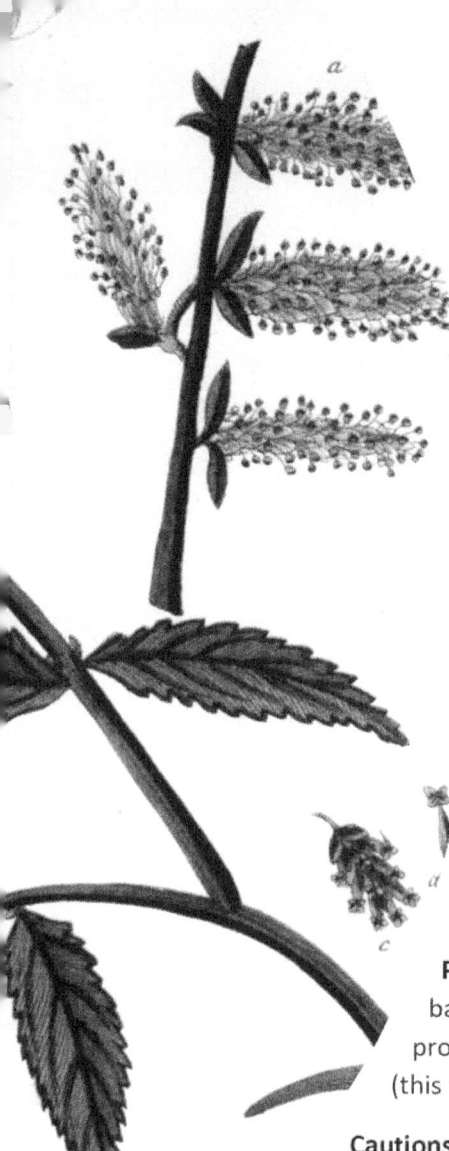

Willow

Latin name: Salix alba

Part used: bark

Indications:

A potent anti-inflammatory herb for the musculoskeletal system. Add it in the recipe for any type of muscle stiffness, arthritis and rheumatic pain.

As a poultice (without cloth), it can be applied directly on wounds and cuts.

Preparation: Grind the dried bark in powder, using a food processor, a grinder or a mortar (this will take time!).

Cautions and concerns: It is best to use the bark from cut twigs, or to forage bark that has fallen on the ground. Never remove bark from a living tree, as it is damaging to the plant's health.

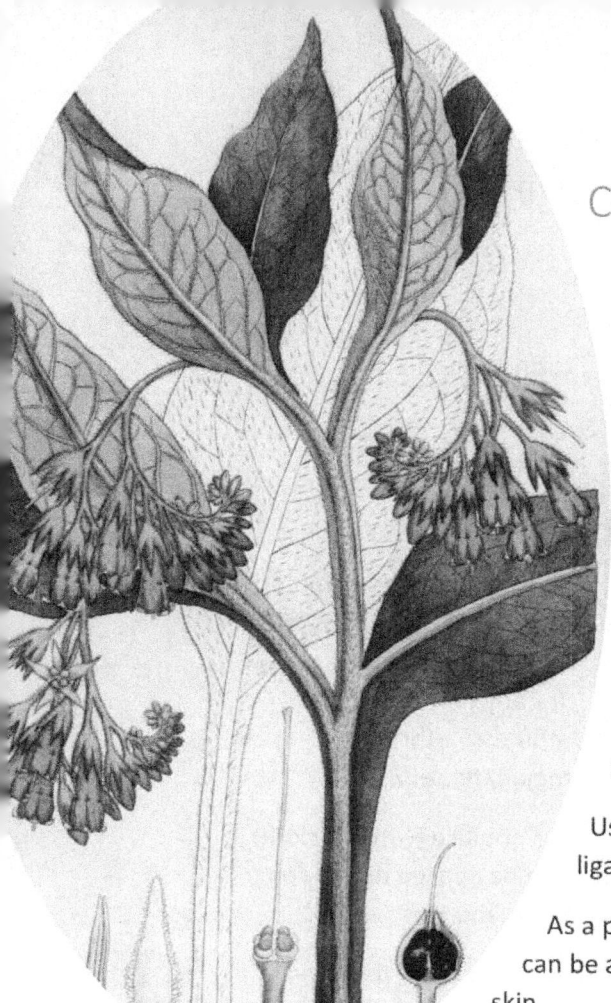

Comfrey

Latin name: Symphytum officinale

Part used: leaf

Indications:

Use it for fractures. Apply it directly on the damaged limb.

It can be added in recipes for arthritis.

Useful for damaged ligaments and tendons.

As a poultice (without cloth), it can be applied directly on the skin.

Its healing action is attributed to allantoin.

Preparation: Mince finely the leaves with a knife. Usually it is used on its own, but it can be mixed with other herbs as well.

Cautions and concerns: Do not apply to broken skin or open wounds. Not to be taken internally. Do not use it daily for more than ten days in a row.

Other Western herbs for packs and poultices

Here are some additional herbs of the Western tradition of herbalism that can be used in herbal packs and poultices.

- **Plantain**. Useful for rashes, scrapes and cuts.
- **Yarrow**. Soothes inflamed skin. The plant also possesses mild anti-inflammatory and analgesic properties.
- **Linseed**. Traditionally applies for boils, inflammation and wounds. Linseed poultices have been used by the army as well.
- **Orange blossom**. They are added in the recipe for their euphoric aroma. Recommended for stress.
- **Artemisia vulgaris** [xviii]. Useful for sore muscles.
- In addition to **bread and cereals**, bran and clay may also be used as a poultice because of its absorbent quality. It is packed into the wound and then covered with a piece of sacking or similar material before being bandaged onto the site of the wound.

A note on Western poultices

It should be noted that in Western herbalism, the word "poultice" means that the herb is minced and placed directly on the skin, usually without heat. (In fact, heat is contraindicated if there is a bruise, a scrape or a cut.) Then, it is secured with bandages, wraps and fabric.

The Thai herbal packs are applied with heat, and their herbs are always wrapped in fabric.

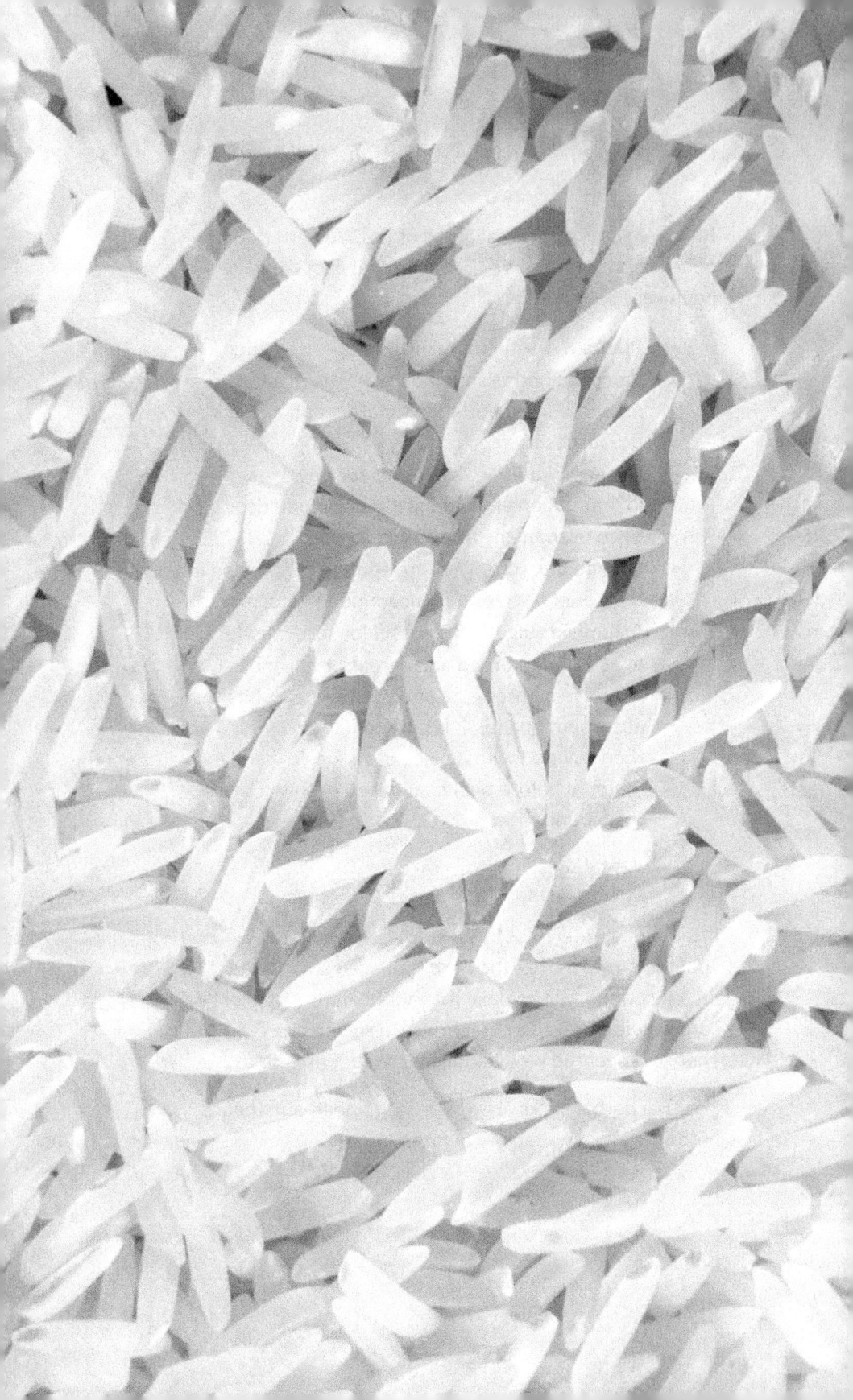

Using sand, salt, stones and rice

It is possible to add sand, stones and rice in the herbal packs. These additions are optional of course. While the herbs possess valuable anti-inflammatory properties, they are soft and porous as a material, and do not hold heat for prolonged periods.

On the other hand, sand, stones and pebbles do not really have these healing properties, but they can retain heat, and this is desirable. When making packs with sand and pebbles, bear in mind that these ingredients will have a much higher temperature than the herbs because of their hardness. Thus, care has to be taken that they are evenly distributed in the pack, and that they will not cause burns.

These are not traditional Thai uses. However, they can be incorporated in recipes with Thai herbs.

Using sand

Collect sand from the beach or from a river. Wash it in clean water, and then clean it through a sieve. Sand is best used when the other ingredients of the herbal pack are grind well, because only in that case it will mix well with the plant material. Otherwise, it will sit on the bottom of your pack, and its heat will not be distributed evenly in the pack.

It is possible to make balls only with sand. These balls will not have a strong anti-inflammatory effect, but they will be very warm for a long time. An additional advantage is that, provided you have collected the sand yourself, the manufacturing cost will be lower.

Moreover, it is super quick to prepare a ball that contains only sand, since there is no chopping involved.

Be very careful not to burn yourself and your client! A ball that contains only sand will be much warmer than one that contains only plant material.

If you do not have access to natural sand, building sand is an acceptable (and cheap) material.

Using salt

It is possible to use natural sea salt, Epsom salts or Himalayan salt. Since I live in Greece, I prefer natural sea salt because it is cheaper! I have also found that its effect is by no way less satisfactory than that of Epsom salts and Himalayan salt.

As is the case with sand, it is possible to either add salt in an herbal recipe, or to make a pack only with salt.

Salt has analgesic properties, and it can be added to recipes for various types of pain. For example:

- Muscle and joint pain
- Headaches
- Sinusitis
- Chronic diarrhea
- Dysmenorrhea (menstrual cramps)

I have found that salt is a useful ingredient in a recipe that contains eucalyptus, peppermint, ginger and camphor.

However, even if you do not have the abovementioned herbs readily available, you can make a ball that contains only salt. Thick salt is a more preferable option in comparison to fine salt, although fine salt is acceptable.

Salt will melt in the hot pack, and will not greatly increase the pack's temperature.

Using stones and pebbles

If you are trained in Hot Stone Massage, you know very well how hot a stone can get! Now consider the fact that a stone massage heater is used at about 40-50 Celsius degrees, while the steamer's temperature is close to 100 Celsius degrees. It is very easy to cause burns on yourself and on your clients, if you use the wrong type of stone.

I have found that adding a small pebble in the center of your pack, suffices. This is how I do it: when you have added all the herbal ingredients on your fabric, add a small stone (about the size of a large bean) in the center. This will increase the temperature satisfactorily.

NEVER make a pack only with pebbles and stones, as it will be too hot.

You can keep the stones or pebbles after a massage session. Discard the herbs, wash the stone with warm water and soap, and save it for your future treatments.

Adding rice in the packs

For me, rice is the less interesting ingredient from this list. It will not add heat, and it will not add remarkable healing properties in the pack. However, it is a cheap ingredient and it is ideal for home use. It can also be used in the spa, and in fact I know that some luxurious spas do use rice in their packs.

You can add rice to your herbal ball in order to increase its volume, or you can make a pack that contains only rice. This can be used in order to soothe muscles. Use only uncooked rice in your packs.

It is possible to use linseed (flax seed) instead of rice. Linseed and rice packs (used actually in poultices and compresses) are very old, traditional remedies, and they are used for various problems.

Discard rice (or any other seed or cereal) after 2-3 days. Keep the pack in the fridge during these 2-3 days. This is for home use only – if you have used the herbal compress on a client, you should discard it after the end of your treatment.

Preparation of herbal balls

Now let's see how we are going to make the herbal balls! First of all, we have to cut the fabric. I 've had some guys in my workshops complaining: "I am going to slice and dice plants and vegetables, wash appliances like the steamer etc., now you are asking me to cut fabric like a seamstress, so what's next? Am I going to wear an apron and dishwashing gloves?" After all, I am based in Greece, where traditional roles of the genders are quite strong.

Just in case - if you are a man and you feel you will become a hausfrau with all that, may I inform you that in the Thai tradition, herbalism was a male business. Of course, now things have changed.

In order to cut the fabric, you will just need good sharp scissors. A rotary cutter is not necessary, of course. Lay your fabric on a hard, flat surface, like a table. Create a 90 degree cut on the fabric (placing it on the corner of the table is helpful for this), and fold it in order to make a triangle. Match it up, so that you'll have roughly a square. You can actually fold your fabric lengthwise in order to speed the process, and cut more squares simultaneously.

The squares you will cut do not have to be precise – that is, it is OK if their sides and angles are not *exactly* equal. However, your fabric *should* resemble a square, otherwise you will not be able to create and tie properly your herbal ball. Moreover, the herbal material will "leak" from your herbal ball if the fabric you cut looks more like a rectangle.

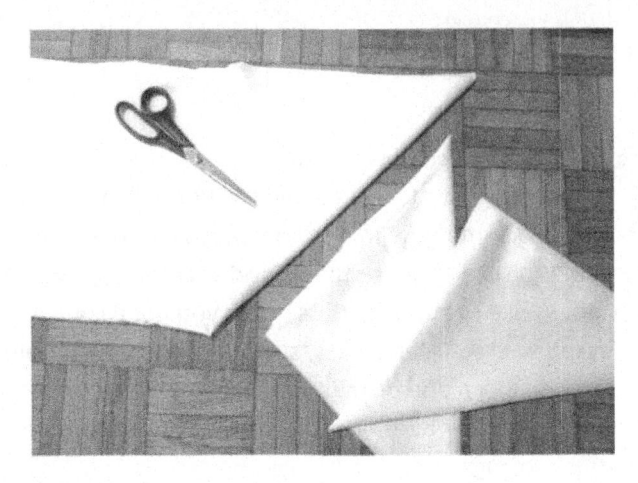

Create a 90 degree cut on the fabric, and fold it in order to make a triangle. Match it up, so that you'll have roughly a square.

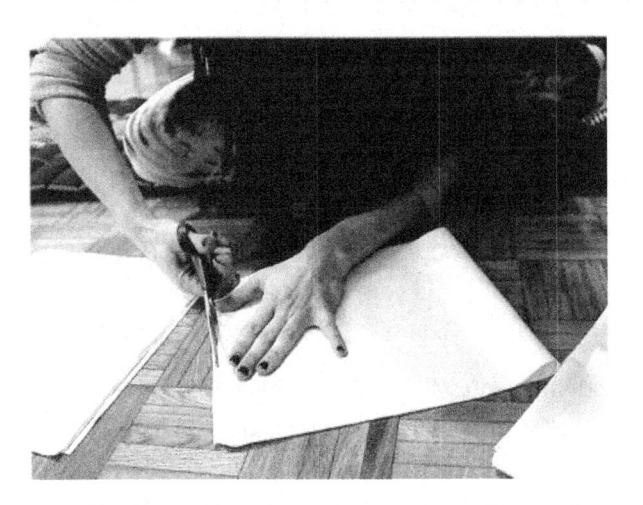

If you fold your fabric lengthwise, you will speed the process, and cut more squares simultaneously. Of course, this is helpful only if you want to make more than two herbal balls.

What are the ideal fabric dimensions for the herbal balls? 50 cm X 50 cm (that's about 20 inches) is a good size for the large herbal balls. Some people like to cut 30 cm X 30 cm (that's about 12 inches) pieces for smaller herbal balls that will be used in facials.

I have found out that the 50 X 50 herbal balls can be used on the face as well, so if your treatment includes work on the body and it is not just a facial, make only this size. You can use a ruler or a tape measure in order to cut the fabric.

28. Large and small herbal balls.

So, how many herbal balls should you make for one professional treatment? Well, you should make at least two.

The idea is that you work on the problematic area with one herbal ball, while the other herbal ball is in the steamer. Then, when the herbal ball starts to become cold, you put it back in the steamer and use the other one. Of course, this process will be repeated many times during the treatment.

If you are using the herbal balls in Swedish massage and you are sliding them on the client's oiled body, you also need two compresses – one for each hand of yours. It is wonderful to make effleurages with the herbal balls.

I know some people who like to work 3 or even 4 herbal balls. 3 is ok, but I think 4 is a bit too much and I do not recommend it. As for me, I always work with two herbal balls.

If you want to apply a hot herbal compress at home, e.g. for a lower back pain, one compress is enough. Just make it, steam it and place it on the painful area. Repeat three times daily, for twenty minutes each time. Keep the compress in the fridge, in a sealed bag.

Methods of tying

Now we will see four different methods of tying and creating an herbal ball.

The key points to making beautiful AND reliable herbal balls are:

- Use the correct amount of herbal material in the correct size of fabric. If you place too many herbs on the fabric, you will not be able to tie the herbal ball properly. If you place a very small quantity of herbs, your handle will be too large, and your herbal ball too small. A small herbal ball means that it will not have the desired therapeutic effect. As a general rule, an amount of herbs equal to a fist, in a 50X50 cm fabric, is recommended.
- Have in mind that finely sliced herbs will result in a tighter compress.
- Make a firm ball, by pressing the herbal material. When the compress is steamed, the herbal material will become loose. Thus, it is good to make a firm compress before steaming it.
- The handle (if you decide to make one – we will see that there is a way to make a very easy compress without a handle) should also be tied firmly and orderly. This prevents the leakage of herbs, and is a key factor for a beautiful herbal ball.

Method #1 – Lazy Girl's Compress

Let's begin with the easy way. This method of tying does not create a handle. Although it is less visually appealing than the other methods, it will result in a reliable compress, which is ideal for home use or for a budget massage therapy or physiotherapy center. It is absolutely suitable for professional use.

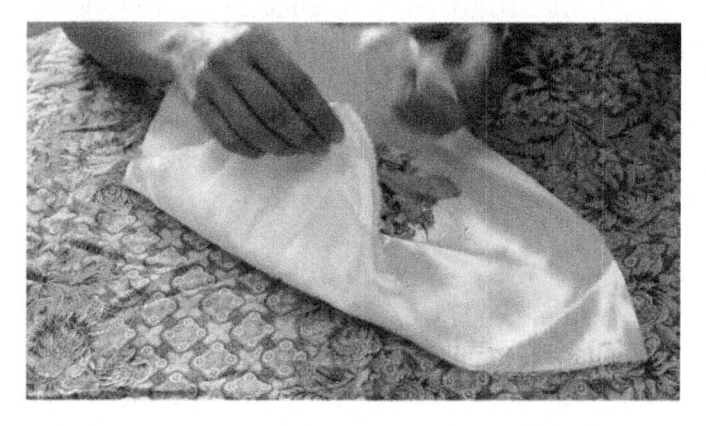

a. Place the herbal material in the center of the fabric. Grasp the opposite corners of the fabric, and make a simple knot. Do not tie it too tightly, neither too loosely.

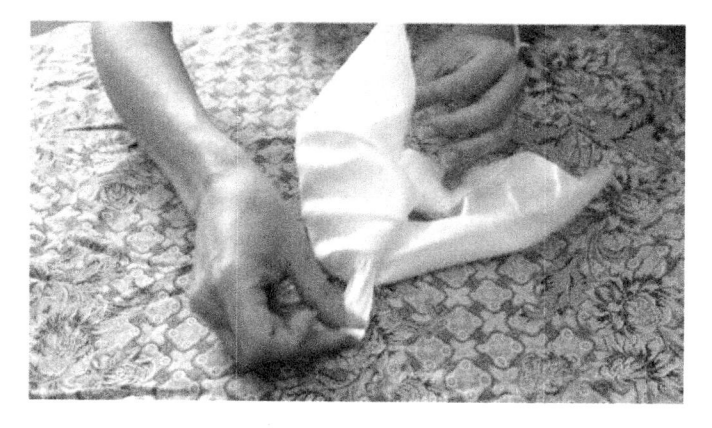

b. Then grasp the other two opposite corners of the fabric, and make again a simple knot. At this stage, you can press (and even hit lightly) the compress against the flat surface, in order to make it firmer.

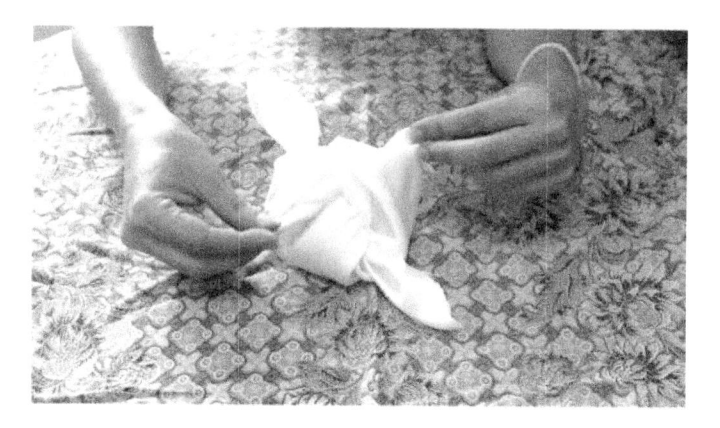

c. Repeat, by making two more knots again, with the opposite corners of the fabric. Tie the last two knots more tightly than the first two ones. Voila! Your herbal compress is ready for steaming and applications.

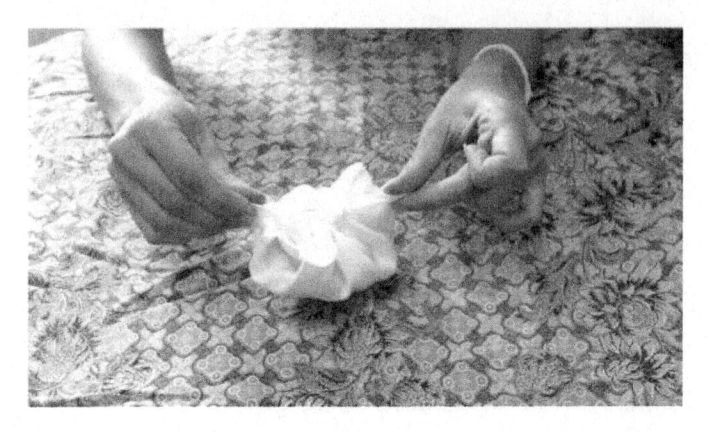

d. This is how it will look in the end. I have done massage treatments with these type of compresses. Just pick the ends of the fabric from the steamer, and you are good to go. The ends will not be hotter than a handle, so there is no concern for this.

Method #2 – Easy & Elegant

This is the easiest method for the production of an herbal ball with a handle. Thus, it is the most common type of herbal balls found in spas. However, generally this type of compress is not sold commercially.

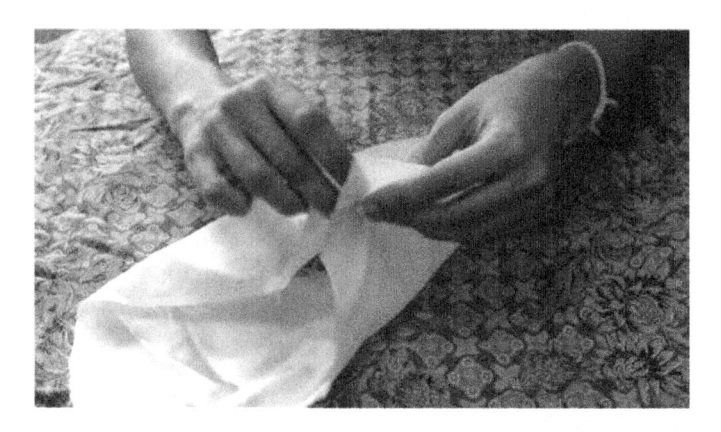

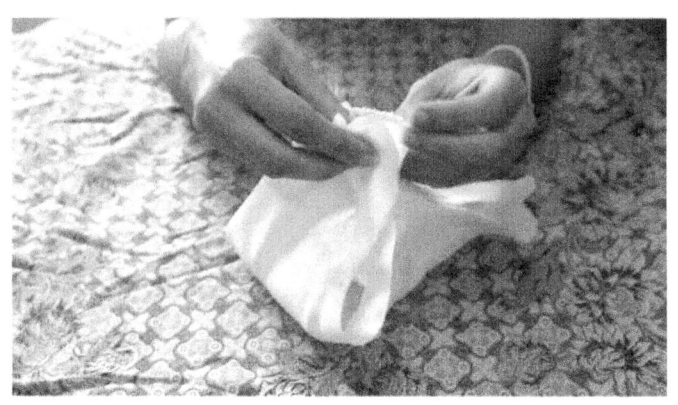

a. Place the herbal material in the center of the fabric. Grasp the opposite corners of the fabric, and bring them together.

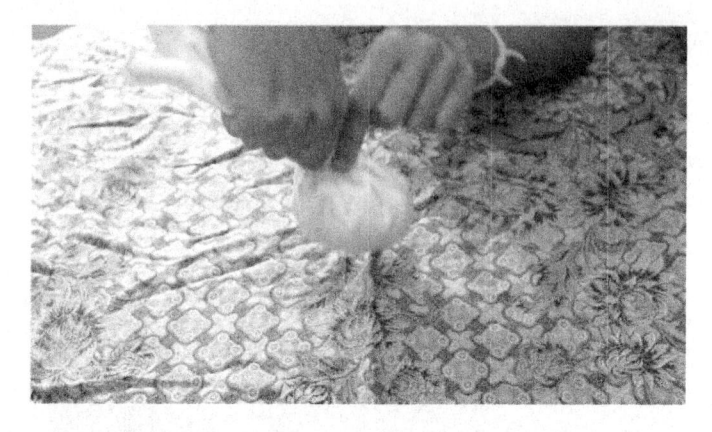

b. Secure the top of the ball with a string. It is recommended to do that with the string you will use to create the handle. For this method, your string should be about 1 meter long (or 40 inches). Leave about 10 cm (or 4 inches) of string, for the final knot.

Some therapists prefer to secure the base of the compress with a small rubber band.

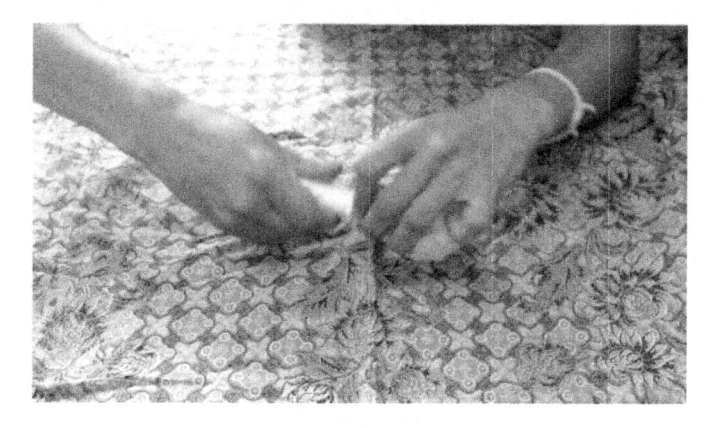

c. After having secured tightly the base of the herbal ball, twist (or fold) the fabric VERY tightly in order to create the handle.

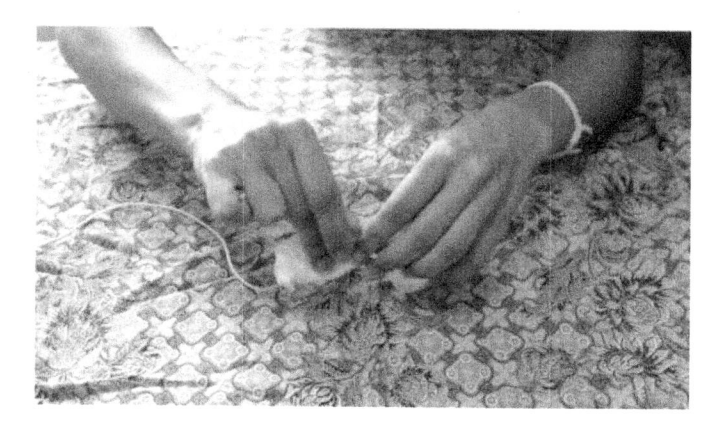

d. Start wrapping the string around the handle. Begin the wrapping from the base of the herbal ball, and move towards the top (= the end of the handle).

The string should be wrapped in an orderly fashion – that is, very tightly. This means that the fabric should not be visible at the handle, at the final result. When you reach the end of the handle, pull the string and wrap it downwards. When you reach the base of the herbal ball, tie a knot with the piece of string you had left in the beginning.

Some therapists prefer to wrap the string only until the middle of the handle, leaving some loose fabric at the top. This is just a matter of a visual preference.

You can see how this type of herbal ball looks, on page 118.

Method #3 – The Rose Bud

This and the next method are a bit more difficult, and require more string. They result in beautiful herbal balls, which are often sold commercially. Of course, they can be used in the spa as well. They are a little bit more time consuming concerning their preparation – well, just 1-2 minutes longer per compress.

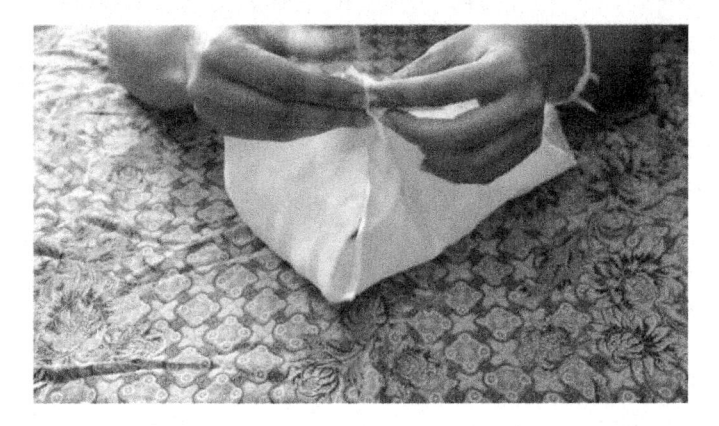

a. Grasp the ends of the fabric, and bring them together.

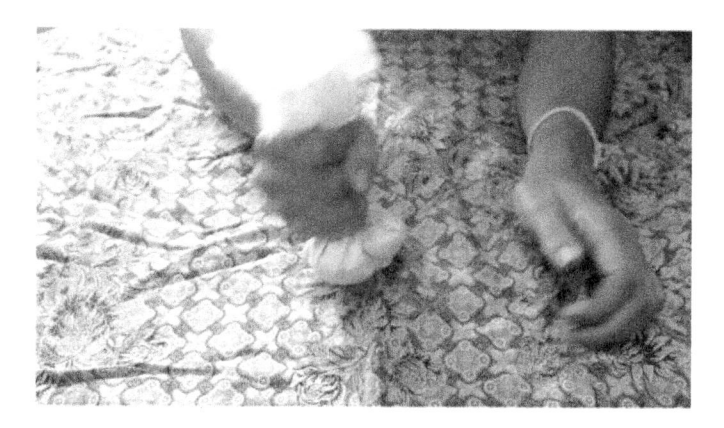

b. Squeeze the herbal material in order to create the spherical shape. Grasp the herbal ball from its base and hit it lightly on your surface, in order to create a firm compress.

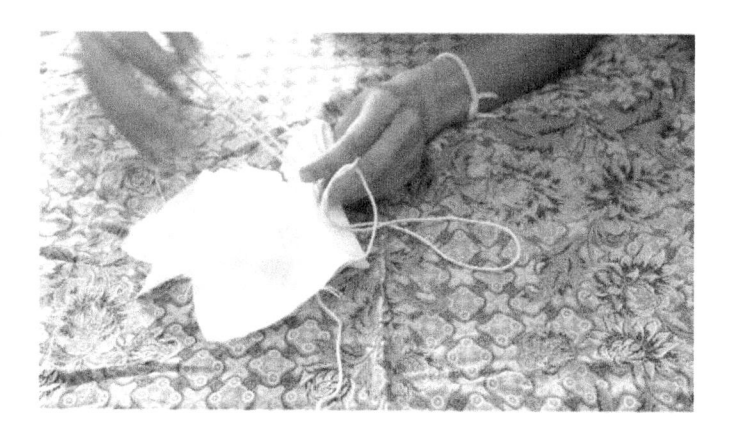

c. Secure the top of the ball with a string. It is recommended to do that with the string you will use to create the handle. For this method, your string should be about at least 1 meter long (or 40 inches). Leave about 10 cm (or 4 inches) of string, for the final knot.

Some therapists prefer to secure the base of the compress with a small rubber band.

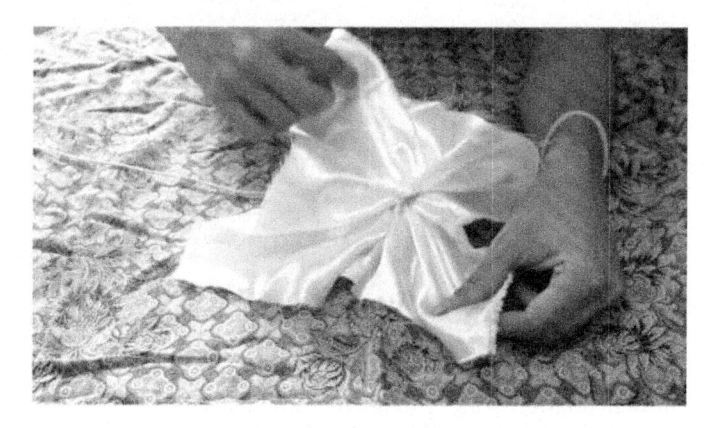

d. Having secured the ball, stretch lightly the fabric and open it, as shown in photo, in order to create the handle.

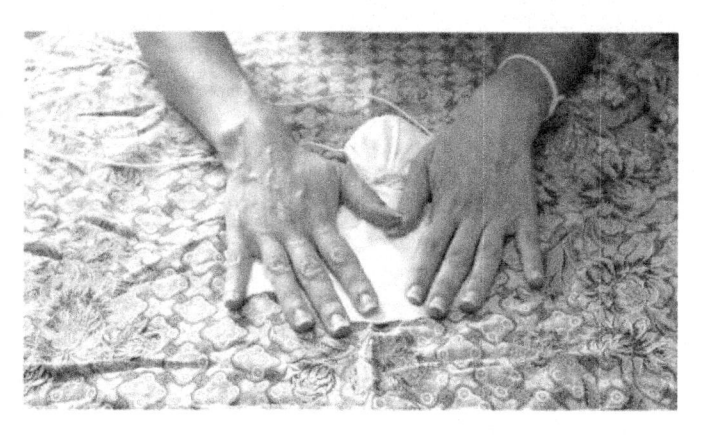

e. Fold the fabric and lay it on your surface. Its shape should resemble an isosceles trapezoid.

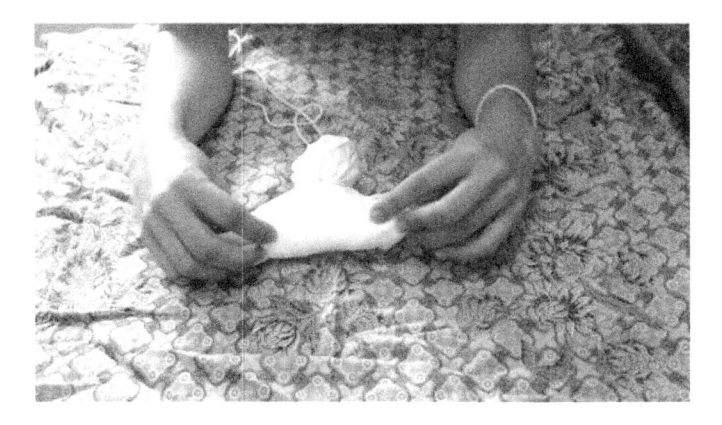

f. Start folding the "trapezoid" tightly, in order to create the handle. Do not roll it – fold it in strips until you end with one large strip.

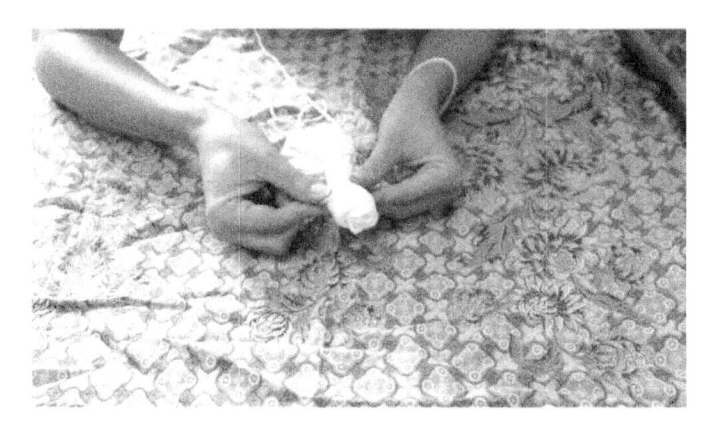

g. Roll this strip in order to create the handle. Then, start wrapping the string around the handle tightly, as in the previous method. Begin the wrapping from the base of the herbal ball, and move towards the top (= the end of the handle). Tie the ends of your string, and the compress is ready! On page 27, you can see some herbal balls made with this method.

Method #4 – The Thai Way

This method of tying results in a very elegant herbal compress. You will need about 2 meters of string – that is, the double amount than that required for the other types of herbal balls.

The following photos were taken in Hang Dong School, in Chiang Mai.

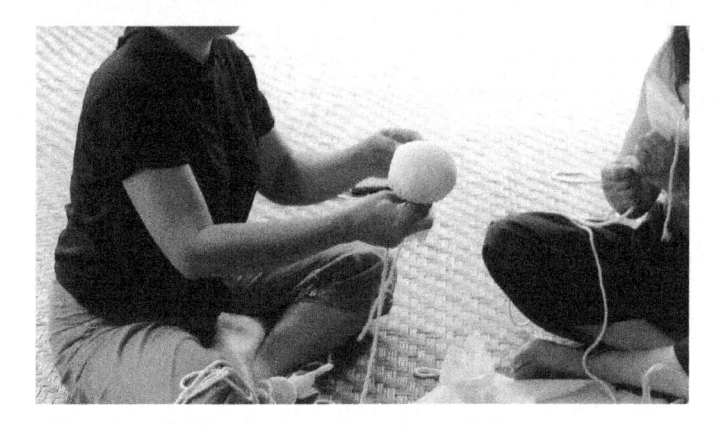

a. As in the other types, start by placing the herbal material on the center of the fabric. Bring together the ends of the fabric, in order to create the spherical shape. Fold the remaining fabric, in order to start creating the handle.

Secure the base of the ball with a rubber band, and tie your string on the base. From this knot, leave about 50cm of string. This piece of string should be folded in the handle, and left "hanging" from the end of the fabric.

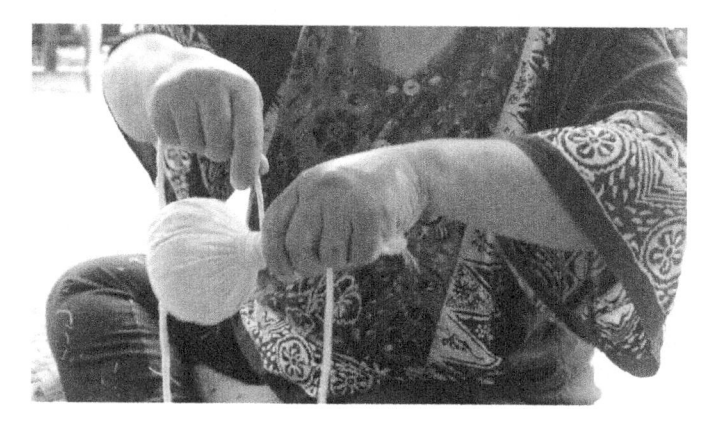

b. Start wrapping the string around the handle tightly, as in the previous methods. Begin the wrapping from the base of the herbal ball, and move towards the top (= the end of the handle). The other "hanging" end of the string should be tucked in the handle. When you reach the top with the larger piece of string, place it parallel to the handle, with its end facing the base of the herbal ball.

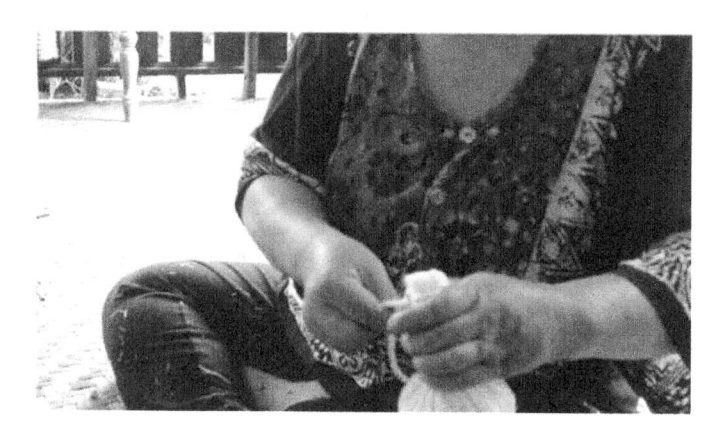

c. Just before reaching the top of the handle, fold the ends of the fabric and place them firmly on the handle. Secure them by wrapping them the "hanging" piece of string.

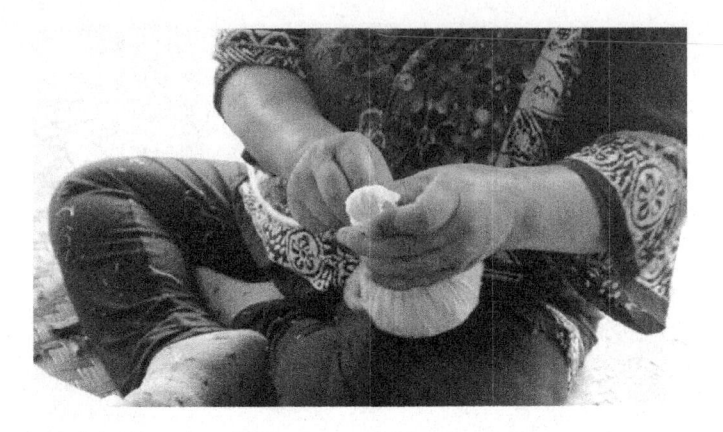

d. Now use the "hanging" piece of string to further secure the handle, by wrapping it around it the handle, in a downwards direction – that is, from the end of the handle towards the base of the herbal ball.

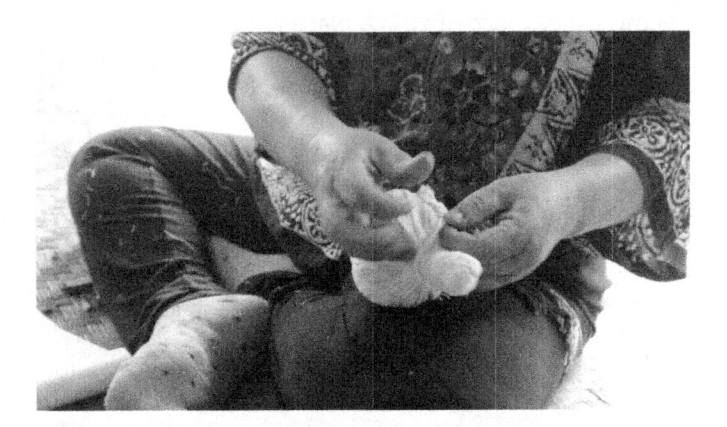

e. When you reach the base of the herbal ball, tie a knot with the two ends of your string.

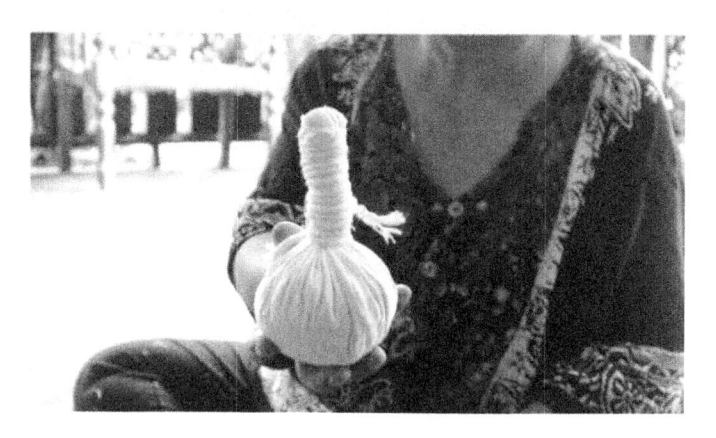

f. Voila! Here is the final result. The handle is 10-15cm long, and actually that's how long it should be in all the herbal ball types.

You can view a free video of this method on my YouTube channel:

https://youtu.be/64uG_NMkXAQ

This video is unlisted, and I am sharing the link only with the readers of my book. Please be considerate and do not share it with other people.

Here's a free, public video on Yam Khang and Luk Pra Kob:
www.youtube.com/watch?v=KQ--KM5Z3Jw
Feel free to share that one!

สถานที่ขายยาแผนโบราณ

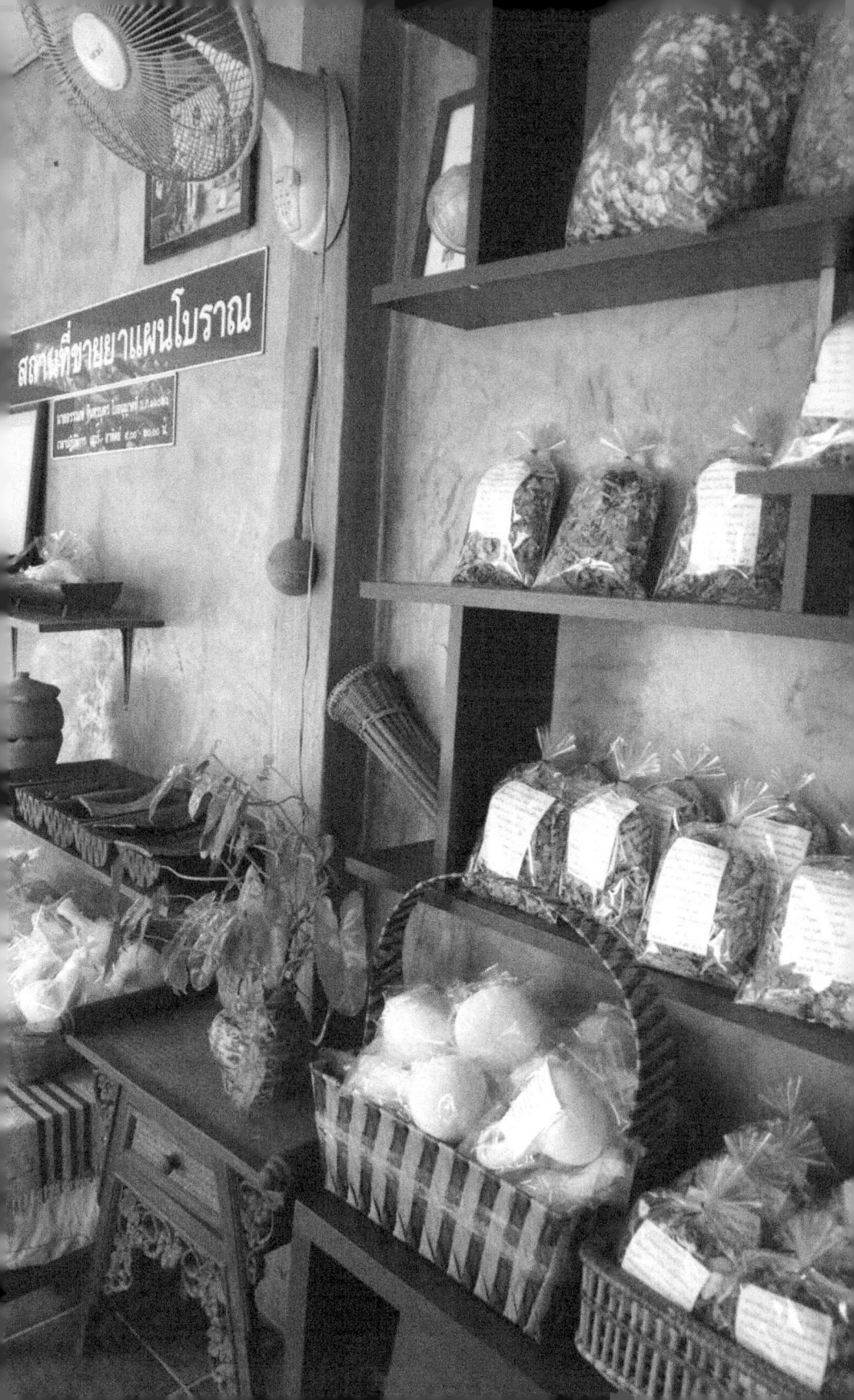

Recipes

Now we are going to see some recipes for your herbal balls. The truth is that there are no standard recipes, and each therapist has his-her own recipes. I will share with you the recipes I was given by two different instructors in Thailand. However, since some of these herbs will be either hard to find or expensive, I urge you to use what is readily available in your area. Anyway, I believe that local products and businesses should be supported – however, this should not become a dogma (in fact, nothing should become a dogma!).

Thus, if you live in the West, it is a good idea to use some inexpensive Oriental herbs, like camphor, ginger and turmeric, and enrich the blend with additional suitable herbs that grow in your area.

29. Thai herbs sold in a street market in Northern Thailand.

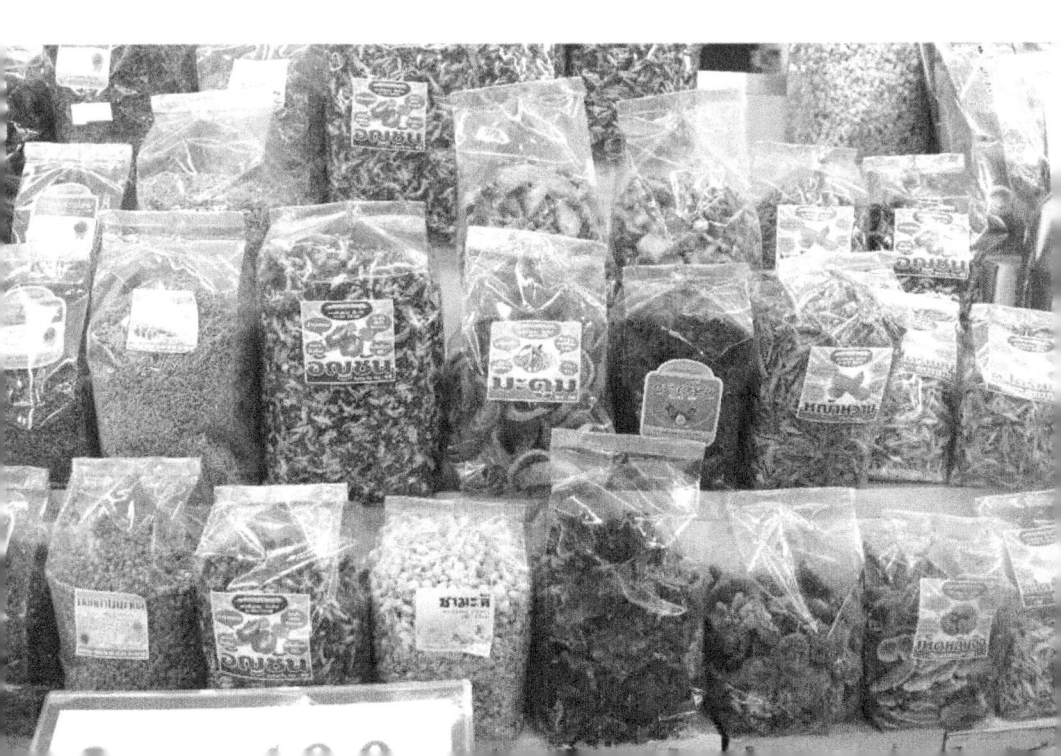

What follows is a general formula I was given in Thailand, with the terms (hot, aromatic, specific) used by my Thai instructor. An herbal ball recipe should contain:

- A "hot" herb (that is, a rubefacient herb).

- An "aromatic" herb – thanks to its fragrance, it has stress-relieving properties and "balances" the somehow pungent, "pharmaceutical" odor of the other herbs.

- A "specific" herb. This refers to an herb that possesses medicinal properties that address the client's health problems (e.g. a potent anti-inflammatory herb, or an expectorant herb).

30. A bowl of Thai herbs which will be added in a herbal ball.

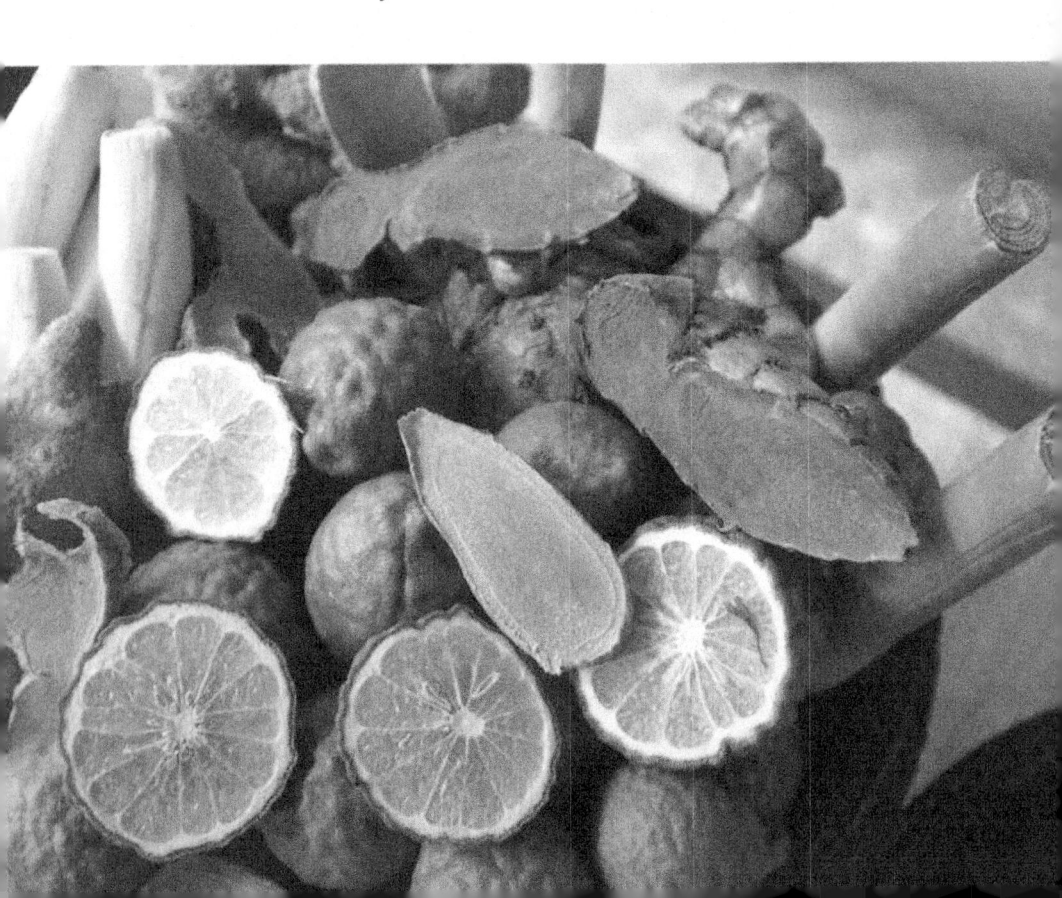

And here is a recipe, according to the previous formula:

- Phlai Ginger (hot)
- Thai mint (hot)
- Kaffir Lime peel (aromatic)
- Eucalyptus leaves (specific)
- Lemongrass (aromatic)
- Tamarind leaves (specific)

There are no strict proportions, although the aromatic herbs should never occupy more space than the "hot" and the "specific" herbs. After all, they are added because of their fragrance, and not because of their medicinal properties. And yes, you can add the other herbs in equal proportions (except the camphor).

There goes one more recipe with Thai herbs, from another practitioner:

- Camphor powder (one teaspoonful) – add it in the end, on top of the other herbs.
- Cinnamon leaves
- Cumin seed (one teaspoonful)
- Eucalyptus leaf
- Kaffir lime peel
- Lemongrass
- Amomum uliginosum (Wan Sao Long leaf)
- Phlai ginger

This recipe, with the addition of Galangal ginger, can also be used in the bathtub or in an absolutely refreshing hammam (steam bath). As a hot herbal ball, it is very effective for muscular pain and tension.

As for the amount of the herbal material that should be placed in the herbal ball, I would say it is about the size of a handful. The only restriction is with camphor powder – never exceed 1-1/5 teaspoonful.

Ehm...now we'll see the recipes I have developed. But before we go there, I'd like to share with you my substitutions (and omissions!).

- Cinnamon leaf: I use bay leaf, as both plants belong to the same botanical family, the Lauraceae, and have similar medicinal properties.
- Phlai ginger (and also Galangal, and Zerumbet ginger): I use Ginger officinalis (the common ginger which is sold in super markets). Also rich in zingiberone and the other anti-inflammatory compounds of the ginger botanical family. Thai gingers are available only frozen, in very few stores, and they are expensive.
- Lemongrass: Although it is generally available, it can be expensive or not readily available. Thus, whenever I do not have it, I use lemon verbena (Aloysia citrodora) or lemon balm (Melissa officinalis). Both herbs are rich in healing aldehydes, as is lemongrass. Plus, I grow them myself!
- Kaffir lime: It is not available where I live. Thus, I use the peel and the leaves of any citrus tree (lemon, orange, bergamot or bitter orange). They have the same medicinal compounds.
- There is no question of finding tamarind leaf, Thai cardamoms or Blumea balsamifera. Thus, I simply omit all these herbs from my blends. Tamarind pulp is available, and I use it.

My recipes

Muscle Pain

- Eucalyptus leaves
- Peppermint
- Camphor
- Turmeric
- Ginger
- Citrus leaf

The particular blend is also recommended for face herbal massage, especially for people with acne.

Fragrant Blend for Muscle Pain

- Eucalyptus leaves
- Bay leaves
- Camphor
- Turmeric
- Ginger
- Citrus leaf
- Lemon verbena (or lemongrass)
- Cumin seed
- Coriander seed

Western blend for muscle pain

- Eucalyptus leaves
- Peppermint
- Willow bark
- Bay leaf
- Cumin seed

...or just comfrey!

It is a good idea to add one small stone in the middle of the herbal ball, for better heat retention. This is recommended for any blend intended for chronic pain relief. Be careful not to use a too hot herbal ball on the face.

Respiratory Problems

- Eucalyptus leaves
- Peppermint
- Camphor
- Ginger
- Jasmine flowers
- Chamomile flowers
- Bay leaf

Anti-stress

- Eucalyptus leaves
- Camphor
- Citrus leaf
- Lemon verbena (or lemongrass)
- Jasmine flowers
- Orange blossom
- Lavender flowers
- Lemon balm

Cosmetic herbal ball #1

- Lavender flowers
- Tamarind pulp
- Lemon balm
- Mallow flowers
- Chamomile
- Jasmine flowers
- Optional: milk powder

Cosmetic herbal ball #2

- Raw rice
- Lavender flowers
- Rose petals
- Orange blossom
- Jasmine flowers
- Optional: milk powder

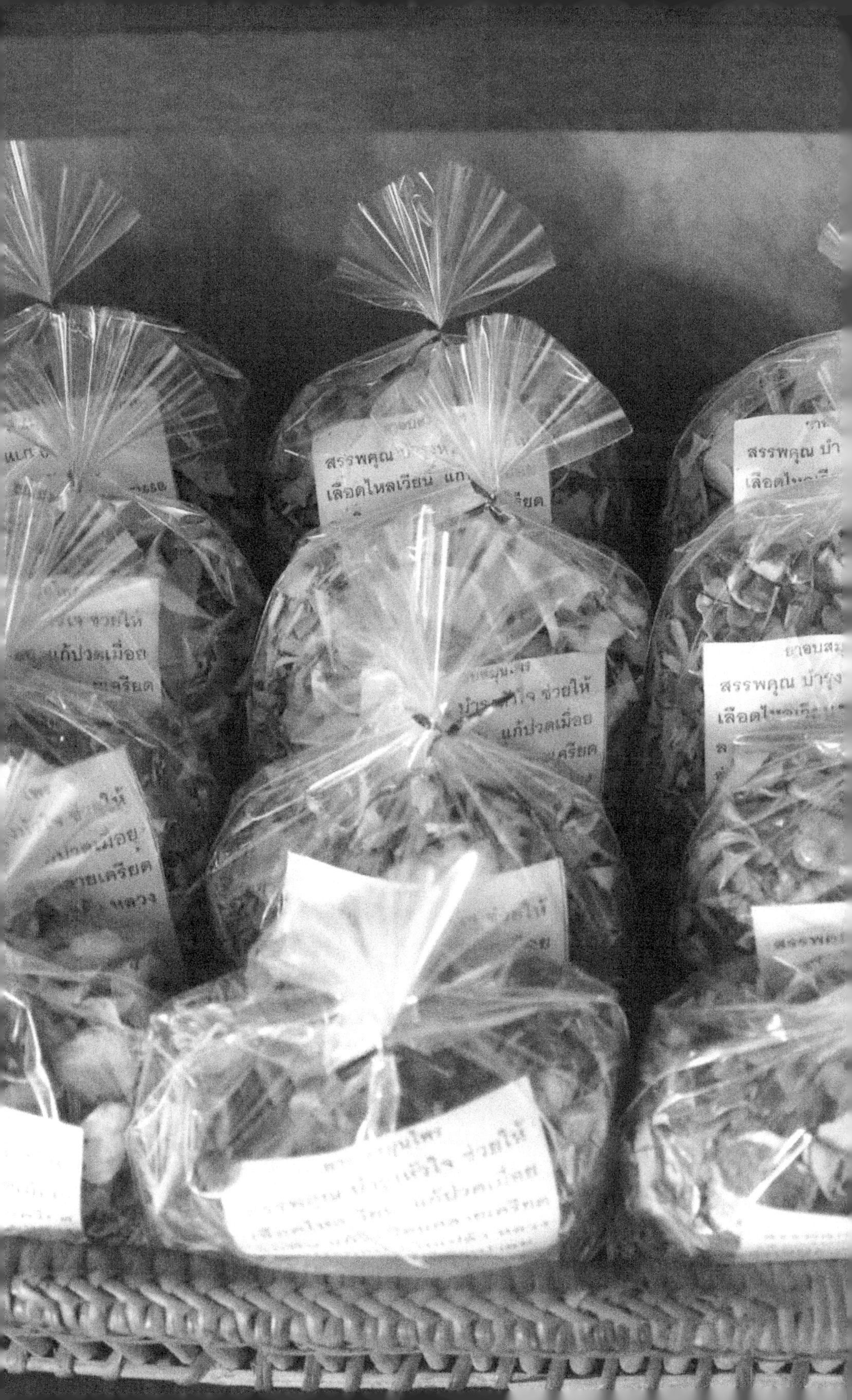
สรรพคุณ บำรุง
เลือดไหลเวียน
ช่วยให้
แก้ปวดเมื่อย

Applications in massage therapy

In this section, I will describe massage techniques with the herbal packs that can be applied in a spa environment.

Here are some basic facts you should keep in mind when handling hot herbal packs. The same rules apply for home use as well.

- Always have in mind that larger packs will retain heat for longer time than smaller packs.
- As you move the herbal balls on and around the body, they lose their heat.
- Do not press too much on the body an herbal ball you just picked from the steamer. It takes about 10-15 seconds until the heat falls to a temperature that is suitable for more static work and deeper pressure.
- When the herbal balls are placed under the body (e.g. under the shoulder area or the lumbar area) they feel much warmer, in comparison to their static application ON the body. Thus, if the receiver feels that the herbal compress is too hot, just move the compress a few inches. Have in mind that the lumbar area is especially sensitive to heat.
- Do not use essential oils – they will evaporate when the packs are placed in the steamer.
- A textbook just cannot describe the heat sensation. Before any professional application, practice on friends, until you master the aspects of speed, pressure and static application.

Using packs in Swedish Massage

The incorporation of herbal packs-balls in a Swedish massage session, will take the treatment to another level.

Some people prefer to soak the packs in warm oil. I have found that using the packs with steam has better results and is less messy.

Techniques

Sliding

In this technique, the balls are slided on the oiled skin, on the back, the legs, the arms and the face. I recommend this technique in the beginning of your treatment, as it will warm the tissues and prepare the body for deeper work.

Just hold the balls and slide them firmly on the body. Work in a quick pace and without pressure when the packs are hot, and more slowly and with greater pressure when the packs are less warm.

Sliding is usually performed with two packs, as each hand holds a pack and slides it on the body.

Stamping

You can do a "stamping" move with the ball, by pressing back and forth its sides on the body. The pace and the pressure are determined by the heat – the faster the pace, the quicker the heat loss. Be careful when pressing on the client's body a hot compress. Start with light pressure when the packs are hot, and apply stronger pressure after the packs lose their heat.

Stamping is usually done in a more focused area - at least in comparison to sliding. Do stamping on a stiff area in order to soften it. Repeat the stamping about 10 times on a spot. Then place the pack back to the steamer and massage the area. Warm the spot again with the stamping technique (10 times), and massage again. Repeat 3-4 times this alternation of packs and massage, until tension is released.

Stamping has excellent results when combined with deep tissue massage and myofascial release work. It makes these techniques less painful and more pleasant for the client.

Stamping can be applied in any part of the body, including the face. It can be done with two packs simultaneously, or with one pack only.

Rolling technique
This is a variation of the stamping technique. Instead of pressing the pack back and forth alternatively, it is possible to roll it on the body in a circular motion. It is used and applied like the stamping.
Remember that the herbal packs lose their heat as you move them.

Static application

Static application of the pack is usually done towards the end of the treatment, or after the completion of the other techniques on the area.

After you have performed massage techniques in combination with warm packs, you can leave the pack on the painful area. I have found that this has excellent results. Leave the pack on the body (or under the body, if the pack is placed e.g. under the back while the client lies in supine position) for as long as it warm.

When placed under the body, the packs can retain their heat for about 10-15 minutes. When placed on the body, they can be pleasantly warm for about 5-10 minutes. Herbal packs should be covered with a thick towel when they are left on the body, so that they can retain their heat for longer periods of time. Remember that larger herbal balls will be warm for longer.

It is possible to stabilize a pack by wrapping it with a cloth. This can be useful for areas where the pack will not stand easily, like the elbow or the knee joint. It is necessary to stabilize a pack on the forehead with a cloth.

Static application of a pack can be done on any part of the body. This is actually like applying a traditional poultice or a compress with Western herbs. Before placing a hot herbal ball on (or under) the client's body, it should be comfortable on your inner forearm, so be sure to check the temperature. Stay close to the client – in case he or she complains, move slightly the packs.

Using herbal packs in Thai Massage

Thai Massage is a dry massage technique, and thus the packs are applied without oil. Moreover, the client wears light clothing during a Thai Massage treatment.

Since, in order to be effective, the packs have to be applied directly on the skin, extra attention and a special technique are needed. Ensure that the client's clothing is loose enough, because the packs will have to be placed under his or her clothes. Place a towel between the client's clothes and the pack, otherwise the client's clothes will be stained and wetted.

Techniques

- Before the application of Thai Massage techniques on any part of the body, grab an herbal pack, and do the stamping technique on the Sen lines that cross the particular area.
- Warm a painful area of the body with the rotation technique, alternating the application of herbal packs with the application of Thai Massage techniques.
- Leave the packs on painful or stiff area and cover them with a thick towel, so that they are not in contact with the client's clothes.
- Place the packs on the Thai acupressure points, before and after the application of acupressure.

The application of hot herbal poultices is sure to take your Thai Massage treatments to another level!

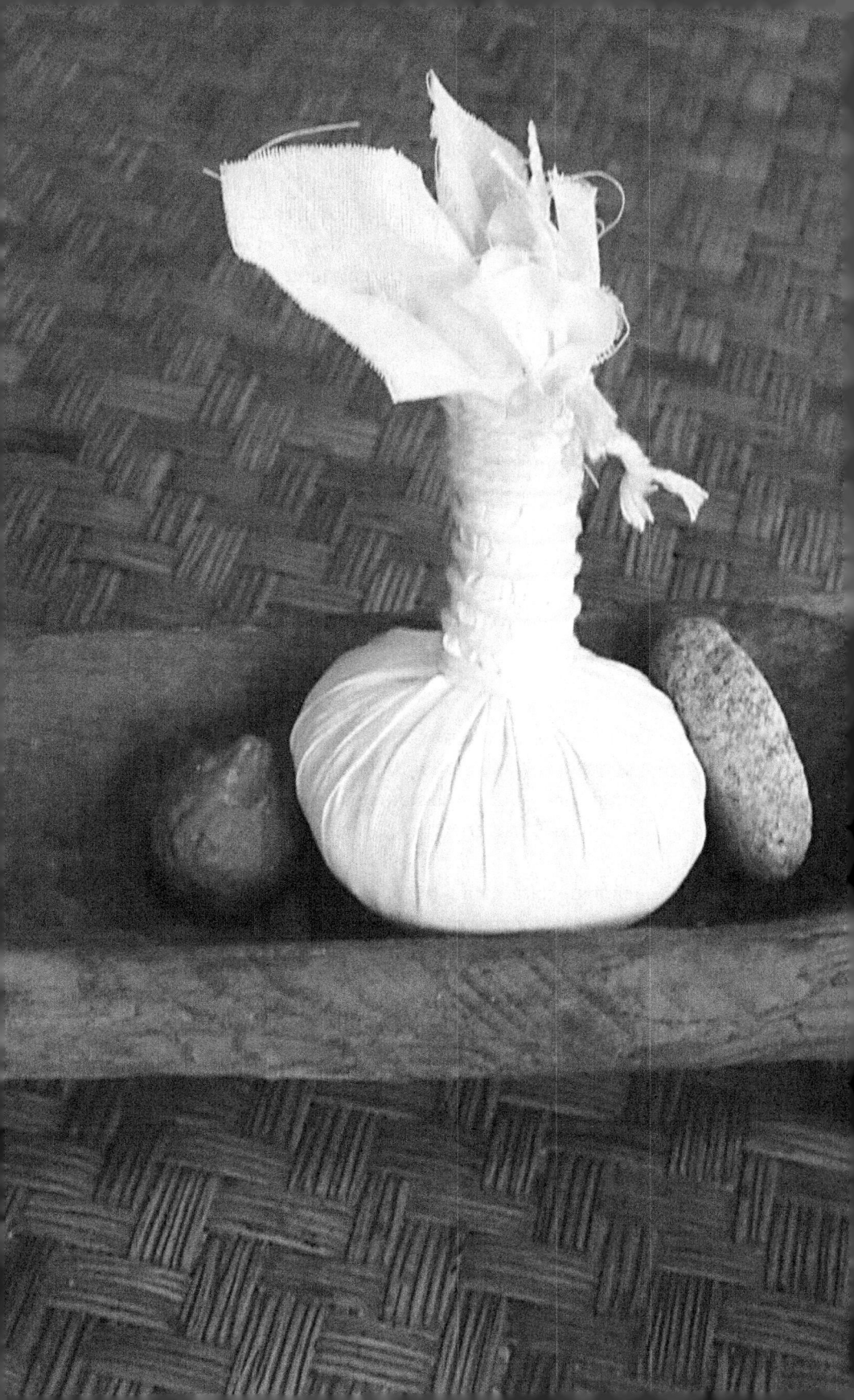

Lay-outs & protocols

In this section, I will describe protocols and lay-outs that include hot herbal packs, for various health problems. My initial training in this was in Mama Lek's school in Chiang Mai, in 2002. As I continued to offer Thai Massage treatments, I developed my own techniques.

However, here's the short version:
Make two herbal balls. Place them in a steamer and heat them thoroughly. Once their aroma emerges (generally after 10 to 15 minutes), they are ready.

Before doing dynamic techniques in the problematic region, warm it with the compress. After kneading and stretching, apply the compress again. Repeat 4-5 times. When an herbal ball is starting to become cold, place it back in the steamer, and use the other, which will be hot. Whenever necessary, use both herbal balls. In any case, once they are thoroughly warm (that is, after 20 minutes of steaming), they will be rewarmed in a matter of seconds when placed back in the steamer.

Before placing a compress on the client's body, first place it on your inner forearm, to check the temperature.

At the end of the session, place them on the temples, forehead, chest, and below the shoulders.

As for the Thai meridians that are mentioned, please refer to the section "Sip Sen – The Ten Lines".

Lower back pain & sciatica

Start by performing suitable massage techniques for lower back pain and sciatica, with the client in prone position. Then, do the "stamping" technique on the Itha & Pingkala Sen on the back, with two herbal balls (one for each hand). Repeat three times, starting from the lower back and ending on the level of the first thoracic vertebra.

Then, place two herbal balls on the lumbar area, and cover them with a thick towel. Proceed to work on the upper back for 10 minutes, and leave the balls on the lumbar area, on the spots occupied by the quadratus lumborum muscle.

Remove the herbal balls from the lumbar area, and place them in the steamer for 10 seconds – this is enough for them to be heated satisfactorily. Place one herbal ball on the sacrum, and cover with a towel. Leave the herbal ball for 5 minutes on the area, and remove.

Conclude your work by sliding one herbal ball right above the pelvis, in order to target the iliolumbar ligament – a common source of lower back pain. In order to do this, start sliding the hot pack from the lumbar spine towards the iliac crest. Repeat 10 times on one side of the back, and repeat on the other side of the back.

Don't forget to ask the client to lie on supine position, in order to work on the abdominal area. I consider abdominal massage work to be a must in any protocol for lower back pain.

When the client lies in supine position, the therapist has the opportunity to apply techniques and mobilizations for the legs – these are always helpful for lower back pain.

If you so wish, you can do the stamping technique with the packs on the legs as well, by pressing the hot packs on the Sen lines that cross the legs.

Use any blend for muscle pain – refer to the "Recipes" section.

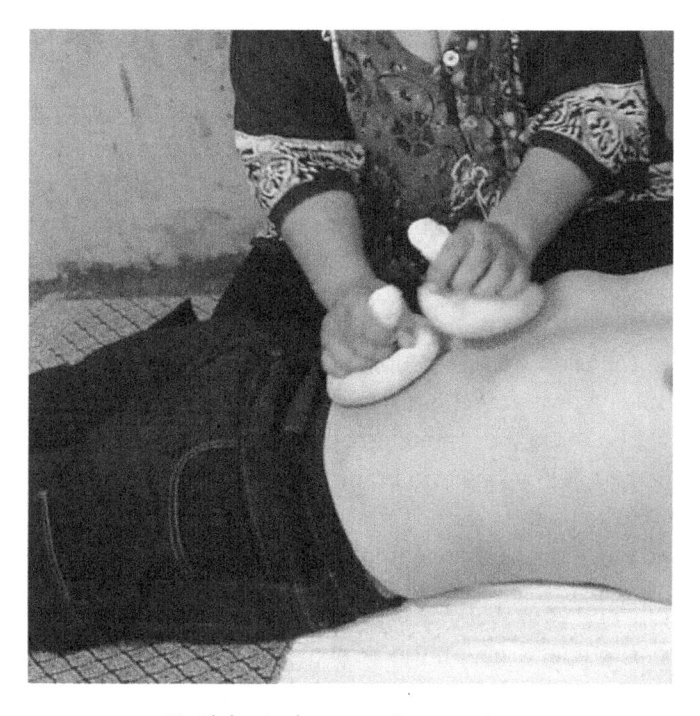

31. Abdominal massage is a must in any protocol for lower back pain.

Neck tension & upper back pain

Start by performing suitable massage techniques for upper back pain, with the client in prone position. Then, do the "stamping" technique on the Itha & Pingkala Sen on the back, with two herbal balls (one for each hand). Repeat three times, starting from the lower back and ending on the level of the first thoracic vertebra.

Then, place two herbal balls next to the shoulder blades, on the level of the 2nd- 4th thoracic vertebrae, and cover them with a thick towel. Proceed to work on the lower back for 10 minutes, and leave the balls on the area. After this time period, remove the balls and place them in the steamer.

Ask the client to lie on supine position. Work on the torso, applying proper techniques and mobilizations for upper back pain. Do the stamping technique on the Kalatharee and Itha & Pingkala arm branches, directing your work from the palm towards the shoulder. Repeat three times, and place the herbal balls in the steamer.

Conclude your work by placing one hot herbal ball under the shoulder area, on the level of the 1st-4th thoracic vertebrae. Let the client lie on the herbal balls for 10 minutes.

In a Thai study, hot herbal compress proved to be an effective complementary or alternative treatment for myofascial pain syndrome in the upper trapezius muscle[xix]. The herbal ball that was used in the study contained Zingiber cassumunar, Tamarindus indica L., Citrus hystrix, Curcuma longa, Cymbopogon citratus, Acacia concina, Blumea balsamifera and camphor, with alternating 20 min heat and surface temperature ≤45 °C for 20 min. The treatment was performed once every three days.

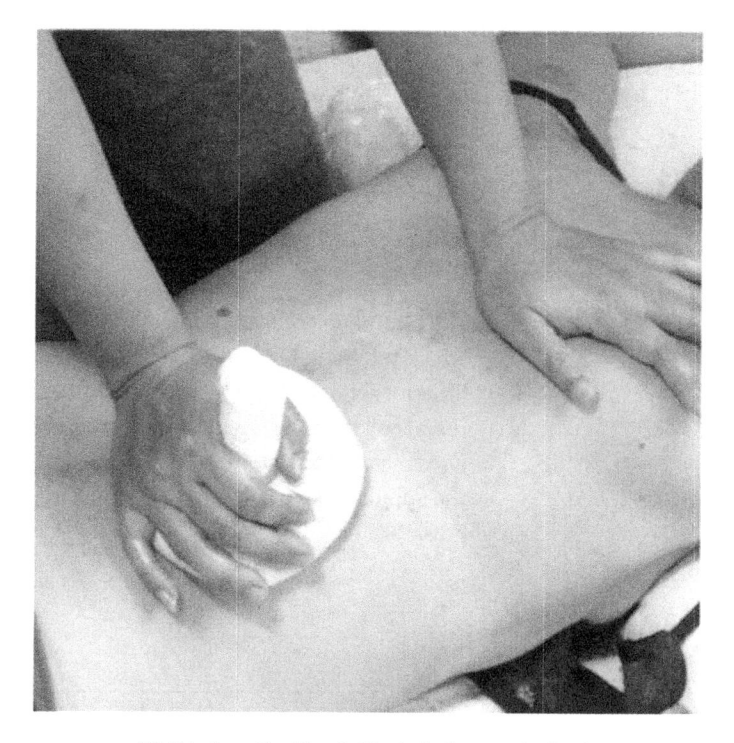

32. Work on the Itha & Pingkala Sen on the back, when treating upper back pain.

Use any blend for muscle pain – refer to the "Recipes" section.

Epicondylitis

Tennis elbow (also known as lateral epicondylitis) is a common injury associated with the lateral epicondyle of the humerus.

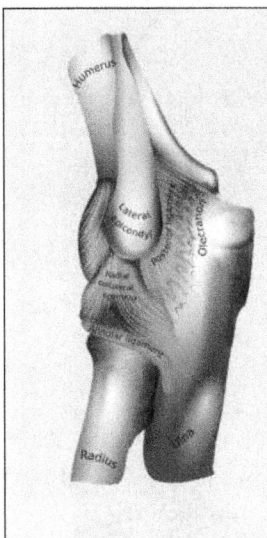

The lateral epicondyle of the humerus is a small, tuberculated eminence, curved a little forward, and giving attachment to the radial collateral ligament of the elbow joint, and to a tendon common to the origin of the supinator and some of the extensor muscles.

Repetitive overuse of the forearm, as seen in tennis or other sports, can result in inflammation of the tendons that join the forearm muscles on the outside of the elbow. The forearm muscles and tendons become damaged from overuse. This leads to pain and tenderness on the outside of the elbow.

Types include:

- Lateral epicondylitis, also known as tennis elbow.
- Medial epicondylitis, also known as golfer's elbow.

Grab a warm herbal pack and perform the stamping technique on the Kalatharee and Itha & Pingkala arm branches. Start from the palm and direct your work to the shoulder. Repeat three times – you need to do this only on the affected arm. Then, place the herbal ball to the steamer.

Grab another warm herbal pack, and start working with the stamping technique on the elbow area. Regardless of which tendon is damaged, work on the outside and on the inside of the elbow. Do 20-30 stamping motions on each spot, and place again the herbal ball in the steamer.

Then, take a warm herbal pack from the steamer, let it cool for about 5-7 seconds, and place it on the affected tendon. You can further secure it with a piece of cloth or a membrane. Leave the herbal pack on the area for 10-15 minutes. During that time, you can either perform massage therapy on other areas of the body, or just leave the pack on the elbow, as you would do with a poultice.

Remove the herbal pack from the elbow, and apply a yellow Thai ointment on the spot.

The herbal pack and the Thai ointment can be used daily, until the inflammation subsides. Orthotic devices can be beneficial, and rest is necessary.

Use any blend for muscle pain – refer to the "Recipes" section. Be sure to add lots of turmeric.

Headaches

Headaches can have multiple causes. A headache may be caused by stress, poor postural habits or hormonal fluctuations. A headache can also be caused by common colds, head injury, rapid ingestion of a very cold food or beverage, and dental or sinus issues. Most headaches are primary, that is, they are benign and are not caused by underlying disease or structural problems.

Whatever the cause, herbal packs can help. Of course, they will be more effective when combined with modalities like Swedish massage, acupuncture, osteopathy and herbal medicine.

Do the "stamping" technique on the Itha & Pingkala Sen on the back, with two herbal balls (one for each hand). Repeat three times, starting from the lower back and ending on the level of the first thoracic vertebra.

Then, place two herbal balls next to the shoulder blades, on the level of the 2nd- 4th thoracic vertebrae, and cover them with a thick towel. Proceed to work on other areas of the back. Leave the packs on the area for about 5 minutes. After that, remove the herbal balls and place them back in the steamer.

If you are doing Thai Massage, proceed with the seated position techniques, and warm the neck and shoulder area thoroughly with the herbal packs. Apply the hot packs before and after each technique.

Conclude your session by "stamping" the packs on the temples and on the forehead. In the end, place the client's head on a pillow, and place one herbal ball on the forehead. Cover the ball (and the eyes, if you so prefer) with a towel, and leave it for 5 minutes.

If you are doing Swedish massage, place the client in supine position, and perform the techniques of the previous paragraph.

I have found that this simple protocol is especially beneficial for cervicogenic headaches – that is, headaches caused by issues on the cervical spine and the soft tissues of the neck.

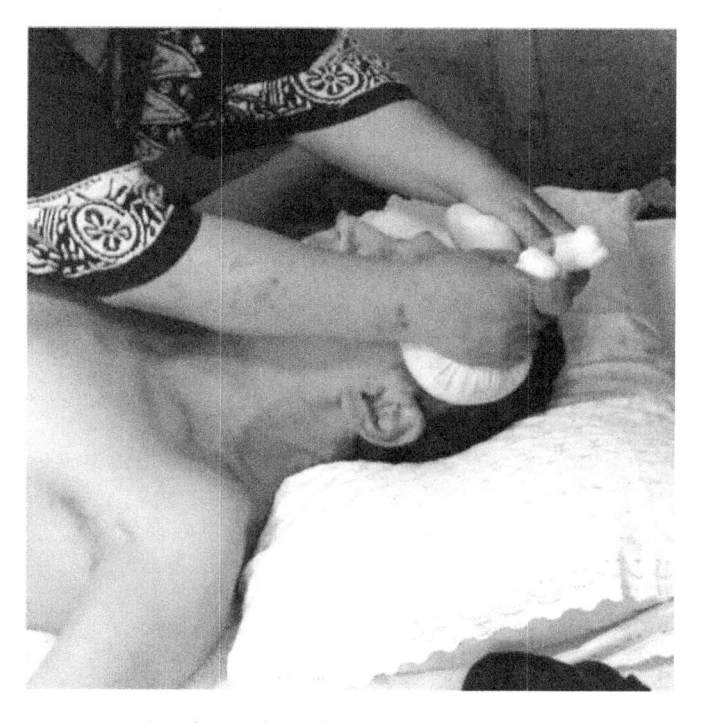

33. Placing the herbal balls on the forehead can be very effective for headaches.

Emotional stress

The application of herbal packs can be very beneficial for emotional stress. Both warmth and fragrance contribute to relaxation.

Begin your work on the Kalatharee sen lines on the arms and the palms, applying the stamping technique. Place one herbal ball on the sternum, and cover with a towel. Leave it there for 10 minutes.

Apply wherever else the client feels tension, and conclude your work by placing herbal balls on the temples and on the forehead.

Use the anti-stress recipe you'll find on Recipes section.

Knee pain

The application of herbal packs can be very helpful for knee injuries and inflammation.

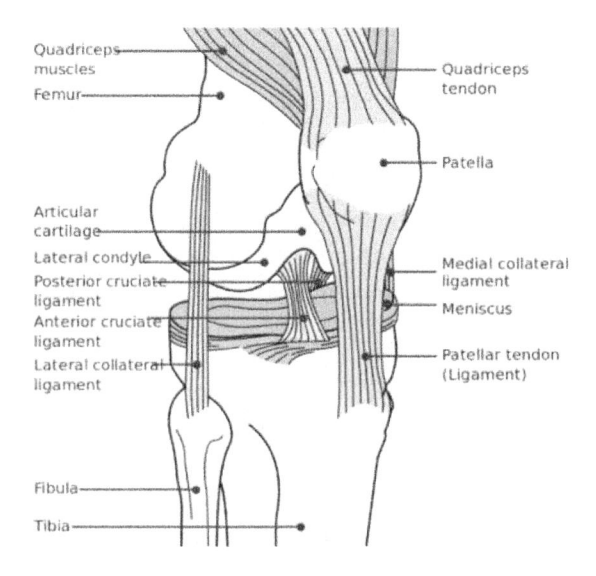

```
Quadriceps muscles
Femur
Quadriceps tendon
Patella
Articular cartilage
Lateral condyle
Posterior cruciate ligament
Anterior cruciate ligament
Lateral collateral ligament
Medial collateral ligament
Meniscus
Patellar tendon (Ligament)
Fibula
Tibia
```

The knee joint consists of an articulation between four bones: the femur, tibia, fibula and patella. There are four compartments to the knee. These are the medial and lateral tibiofemoral compartments, the patellofemoral compartment and the superior tibiofibular joint. The components of each of these compartments can suffer from repetitive strain, injury or disease.

Knee pain is often caused by injured ligaments, a meniscus injury, or osteoarthritis. Of course, during the acute phase of any knee injury (in fact of any injury), the RICE (rest, ice, compression and elevation) protocol should be applied. During the chronic phase, the heat, in combination with the healing properties of the medicinal plants of the herbal ball may be very beneficial.

Knee pain can also occur because of muscle imbalances and tightness, a weak quadriceps muscle or alignment issues of the legs. In these cases, massage therapy could be of great benefit, and the application of the warm herbal packs will greatly enhance any treatment.

Start your treatment by stamping thoroughly the herbal pack on all the Sen lines of the leg. Then, apply stamping motions around the knee joint, and on the patella. Tie the warm herbal pack around the knee with a piece of cloth and leave it on the painful spot for 10-15 minutes. Remove and apply yellow Thai ointment on the painful spot, on the patella and on the popliteal fossa. Remember to always bend the knee before applying an herbal pack on the popliteal fossa.

The client should apply herbal packs on the affected area 2-3 times daily, until the inflammation and the pain subside. Use any blend for muscle pain – refer to the "Recipes" section. Be sure to add lots of turmeric.

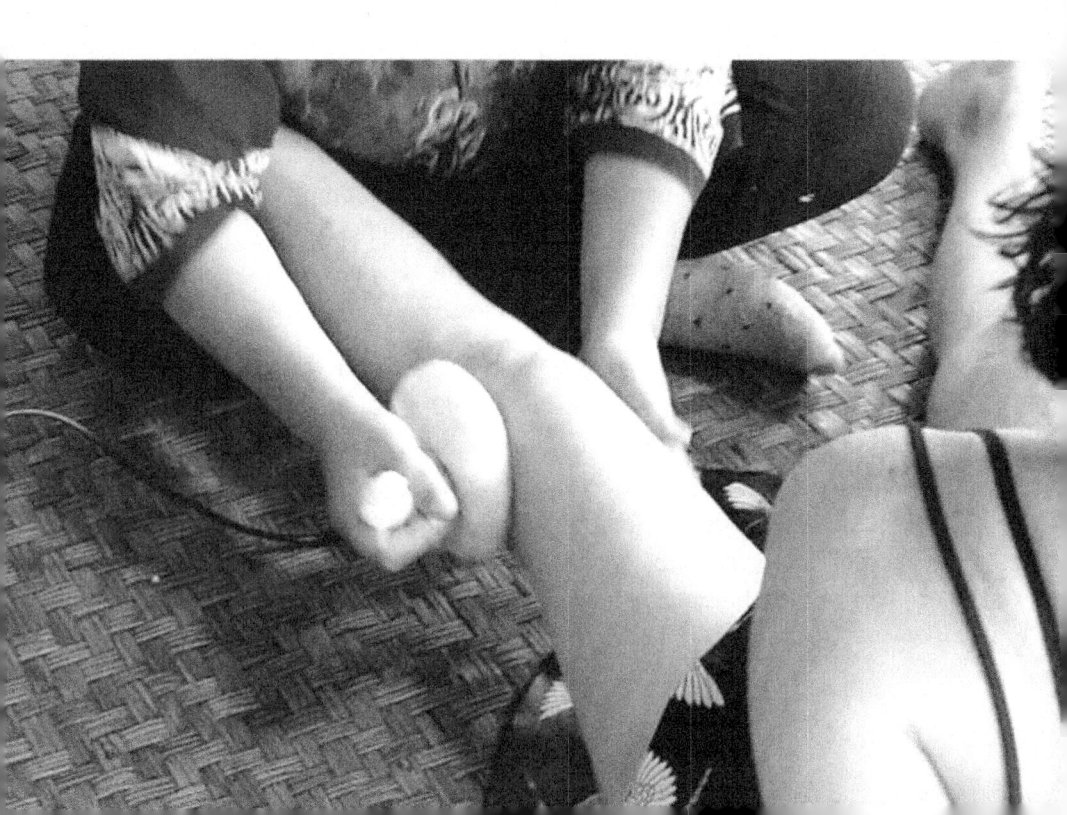

Dysmenorrhea

For dysmenorrhea, I have found that static application works best. Place the herbal balls on the lumbar area (use two – one for each side of the back), and then on the lower abdominal region. Leave them for at least 10-15 minutes in each position.

This is best done a few days before the onset of the period. The heat may induce heavy bleeding, and thus the application of hot herbal balls is not recommended during menstruation.

The therapist may give the compresses to the patient, and instruct her on their use at home. In fact, they can be used daily.

Of course, we are talking about primary dysmenorrhea. Painful menstrual cramps that result from an excess of prostaglandin release are referred to as primary dysmenorrhea. Primary dysmenorrhea usually begins within a year or two of menarche, typically with the onset of ovulatory cycles. Pain results from ischemia and muscle contractions. Spiral arteries in the secretory endometrium constrict, resulting in ischemia to the secretory endometrium. This allows the uterine lining to slough off. The application of herbal compresses on the area stimulates blood flow and has a definite analgesic effect.

Secondary dysmenorrhea is the diagnosis given when menstruation pain is a secondary cause to another disorder, like endometriosis and uterine fibroids. Herbal balls can still be used in these cases, although they will bring only temporary relief.

The packs should contain analgesic and warming herbs, like ginger, camphor and mint. If you so wish, you may add some Western herbs like calendula and chamomile.

Chronic breathing disorders

The application of hot herbal packs is very beneficial for any chronic respiratory ailment. It soothes the bronchi and decongests the entire respiratory system. This is accomplished both because of the heat and the expectorant properties of the herbs.

Do the "stamping" and "rolling" technique on the Itha & Pingkala Sen on the back, with two herbal balls (one for each hand). Repeat three times, starting from the lower back and ending on the level of the first thoracic vertebra.

Then, place two herbal balls next to the shoulder blades, on the level of the 2nd- 4th thoracic vertebrae, and cover them with a thick towel. Apply massage and / or bodywork techniques on the lower spine for 5-10 minutes, and place the herbal packs back in the steamer. Then, since chronic respiratory ailments can often be manifested on the structural level as well, apply mobilizations on the thoracic spine. Many of these mobilizations could be similar to those applied for kyphosis.

Then, grab one herbal pack from the steamer, and place it on the sternum. Work on the trunk and the arms, and then place the herbal pack again in the steamer.

Conclude the treatment with applications (stamping, rolling and static) of the warm herbal packs on the face. Press them on the forehead and on the cheeks.

Give two herbal packs to the client, and instruct him/her to use them at least twice a week. The packs should contain expectorant herbs like eucalyptus, ginger, camphor and mint.

Common cold & flu

This is mostly for family use. Massage is contraindicated during the acute phase of any infection anyway.

Just place one hot herbal pack on the sternum. Use another pack for work on the face – apply it on the forehead and on the cheeks. It is recommended to apply it two or three times daily, until the flu or cold subsides.

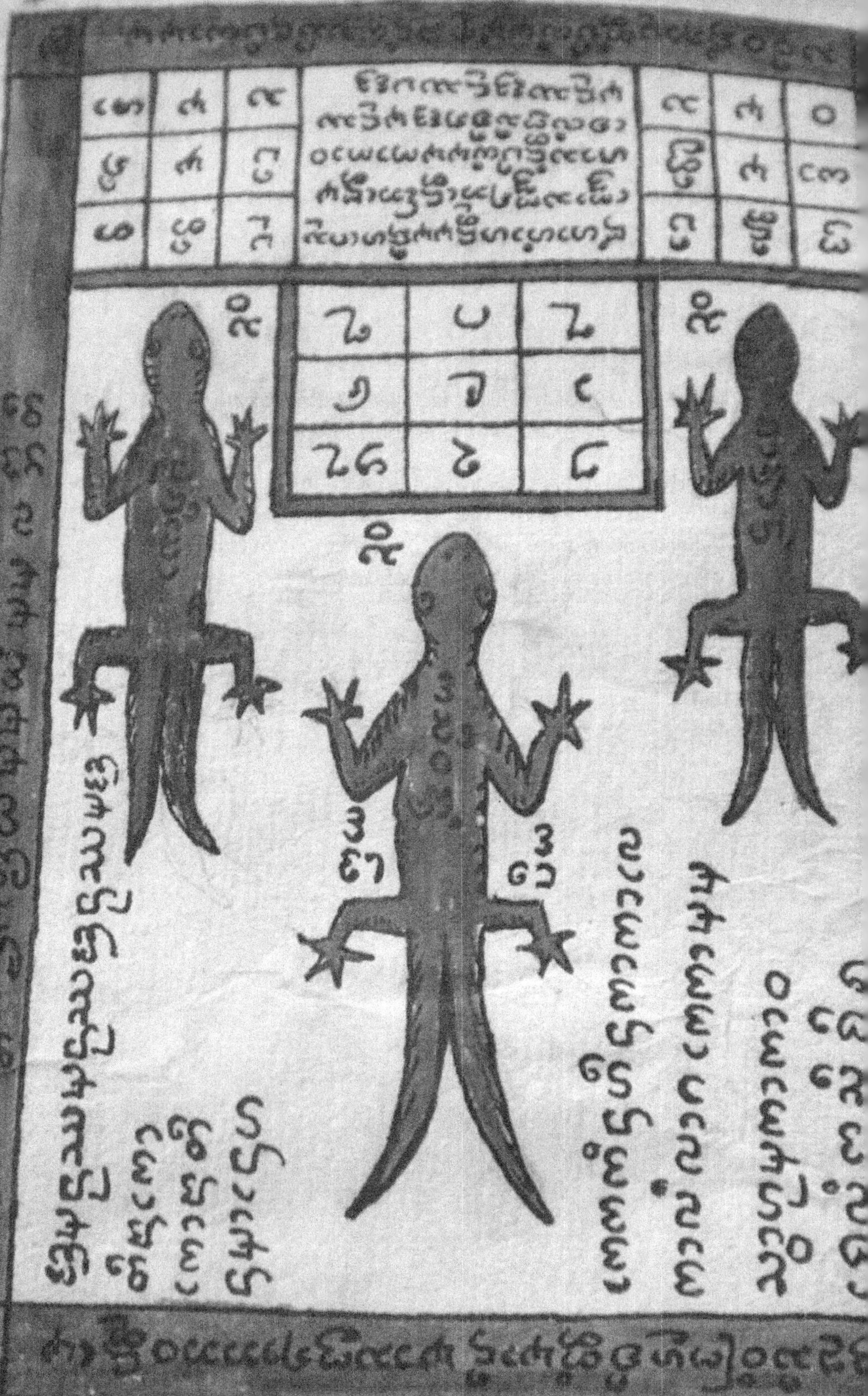

Sip Sen – The Ten Lines

In the Thai language, sen means "line". The Thai meridians are called Sen, and in massage therapy, ten basic "lines" are used (sip means "ten"). [2]

The sen have more similarities with the Ayurvedic nadi, than with the Chinese meridians. The sen do not correspond to specific organs, like the Chinese meridians, and are indicated for problems that may occur across their course. Each sen has some acupressure points.

Sen work is called jap sen, and it is done in 5 steps:

- Stretching (opening the line)
- Walking with palms (warming the line)
- Walking with thumbs (working on specific lines and points)
- Walking with palms (warming the line)
- Stretch (opening the line).

According to the traditional protocol, the therapist should start working upwards all sen lines – that is, from the feet towards the head, and from the hands towards the heart. Then, he should return to the starting point. Bear in mind that there may be some differences to this protocol, depending on the school.

It is not necessary to work all the lines in one session, and it is not necessary to work on the whole course of a line. Jap sen should be applied after training with a qualified teacher.

---

[2] This section contains material from my book "Thai Table Massage".

There are many sen lines crossing the legs. There are three lines on the outer surface of the leg, and 3 in the interior.

These are the lines that run on the outer leg:

1st line: Itha or Pingkala
2nd line: Sahatsarangsi or Tawaree
3rd line: Itha or Pingkala

These are the lines that run on the inner leg:

1st line: Sahatsarangsi or Tawaree
2nd line: Kalatharee
3rd line: Itha or Pingkala

My instructors in Thailand used to say that a Sen line can have one of three colors: white (corresponds to nerves), red (corresponds to arteries), or black (corresponds to veins).

Work on the Sen lines can be used to "open" deeper levels of the body. According to Thai medicine, the human body has five levels:

1. Epidermis (the top layer of the skin).
2. Subcutaneous tissue (also known as the hypodermis or superficial fascia).
3. Sen lines
4. Bones
5. Organs

Now, let's have a look at the Sen lines – the Thai meridians.

1, 2. Itha & Pingkala sen

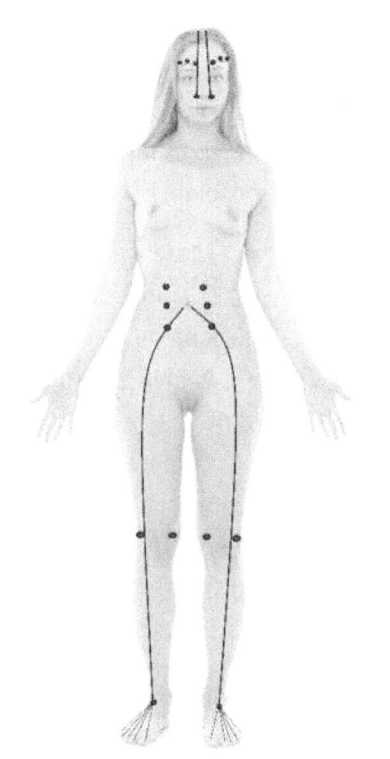

Itha originates from the navel and descends the anterior part of the left thigh, forming the first external line. Then it turns outwards on the left knee, and then follows an upward course between the heads of the posterior thigh muscles, forming the third inner line. It continues its course next to the spine, passes from the scalp and the forehead, and finally ends on the left nostril.

Pingkala follows the same path, but on the right part of the body.

These meridians also have sub-branches.

There is a sub-branch that continues until the toes of the dorsal aspect of the foot, and another that run between the heads of the gastrocnemius muscle (starts below the knee joint).

Also, in the upper part of the thoracic spine, there is another sub-branch, which passes next to the scapula, crosses the anterior surface of the arm and the dorsal surface of the hand, and ends on the fingertips.

Finally, there is a sub-branch above each eyebrow.

Another sub-branch starts from the hip bone and runs down to the ankle, forming the third outer energy line of the leg.

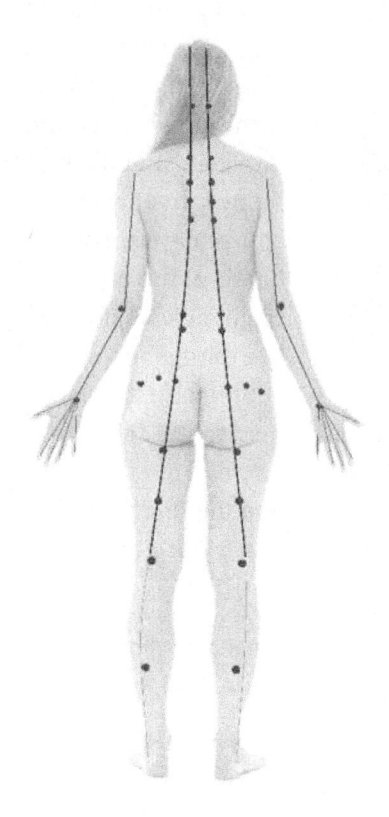

Work on the Itha and Pingkala for these problems:

- Muscle aches (back pain, sciatica, neck pain).
- Pain in the knee joint.
- Carpal tunnel syndrome (work on the arm points shown on the photo).
- Sinusitis (work the points on the face).
- The six points on the belly are used for digestive problems (refer to the section of abdominal techniques for the procedure), and for lower back pain.

These sen are connected to the sense of smell.

3. Sumana Sen

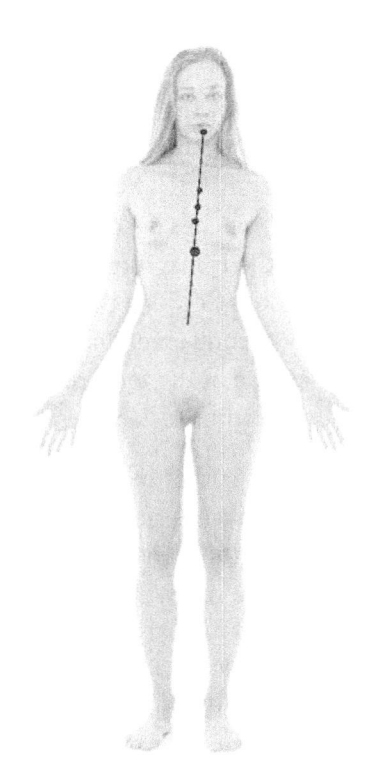

Sumana Sen originates from the navel, crosses the trunk, and ends at the root of the tongue. It is connected to the sense of taste.

Work on Sumana Sen for disorders related to the respiratory system, and the mind (stress, arrhythmias, etc).

The point below the xiphoid process is used for digestive disorders (dyspepsia, gastroesophageal reflux, etc.)

The points on the sternum are used for breathing problems.

The point below the lips is used for nausea.

The point at the root of the tongue is only used when we want to eliminate some toxic substance from the body via emesis. In order to activate it, the finger is inserted into the oral cavity (needless to say, never do this at a client!).

4. Kalatharee Sen

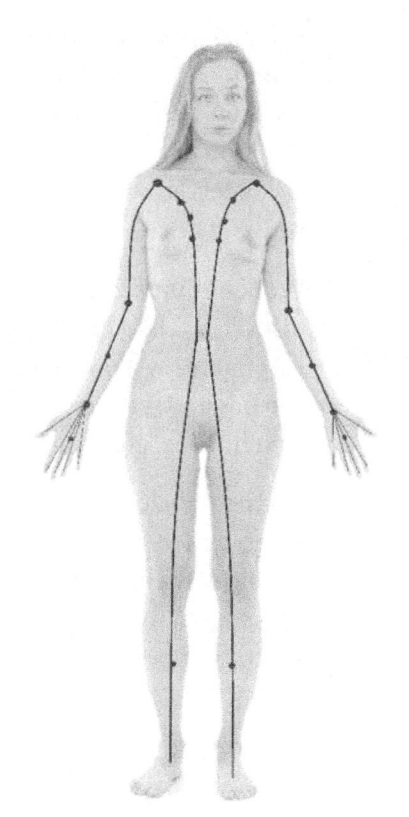

Kalatharee Sen originates from the navel and is divided into four major branches: two branches descend on the trunk, run on the legs (forming the second inner line) and end at the toes, on the plantar surface.

The other two branches run upwards on the trunk, cross the arm (between the ulna and radius) and end on the fingertips, on the palmar surface.

Kalatharee Sen is used for problems in the arms and legs (pain, weakness, numbness, muscle aches, etc.). However, it is also the main sen indicated for arrhythmias and disorders of the nervous system.

Kalatharee Sen is connected to the sense of touch.

The points of the legs are shown in the illustration.

One is located three fingers below the knee, while the other is next to the ankle.

Points on the arms and hands:

The first point of the arm is lateral and superior to the sternum at the lateral side of the first intercostal space.

There is a second point, located in the center of the arm.

The third point is located is located on the transverse crease of the elbow, and it is indicated for tennis elbow.

The fourth point is located at the center of the forearm.

There is also a fifth point on the wrist joint, in the middle of the transverse crease of the wrist. It is indicated for wrist pain, and also for stress and palpitations.

5, 6. Sahatsarangsi & Tawaree Sen

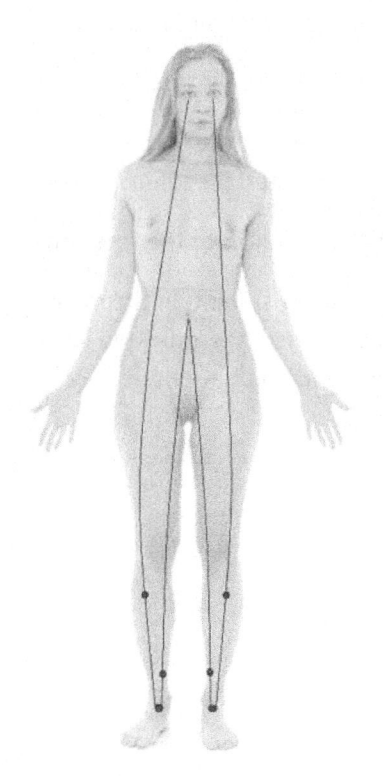

Sahatsarangsi Sen originates from the navel, descends at the inner surface of the left leg, forming the first inner line. Then it turns on the left ankle, forming the second outer line, and runs upwards to the neck. It ends below the left eye.

Tawaree Sen follows the same path, but on the right part of the body.

Both Sen are connected to the sense of sight.

These two sen are used for leg and eye problems. If there is an eye problem, work on the sen that runs on the opposite leg (e.g. if there is a problem on the left eye, work on Tawaree sen).

The first point is located is located four finger widths down from the bottom of the patella, along the outer boundary of the shin bone. Use it for pain on the legs.

The second point is on the dorsum of the foot, at the midpoint of the transverse crease of the ankle joint. It is indicated for ankle pain.

7. Nantakawat Sen

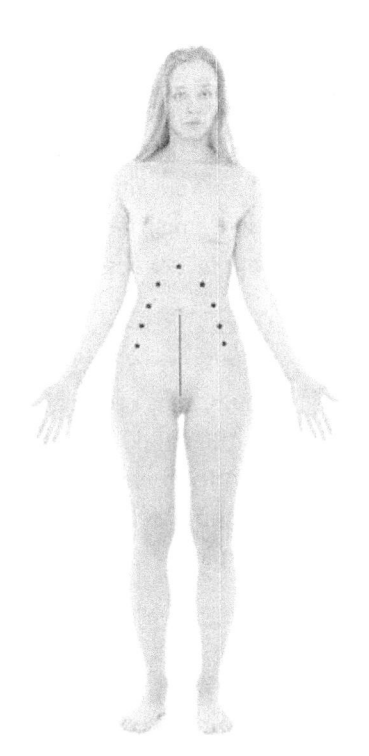

Nantakawat Sen originates from the navel and is divided into two branches.

The first is called Sukumang and ends at the anus, while the second is called Sikinee and ends at the urethra.

This Sen controls the absorption of food, the transformation of liquids and the elimination of waste substances from the body.

Nantakawat Sen is mainly associated with the processes of urination and defacation.

Generally, it is used for digestive problems (constipation, irritable bowel syndrome, etc.).

In cases of constipation work in a clockwise direction, while in cases of diarrhea work anticlockwise, on the 9 points shown on the illustration.

8, 9. Lawusang & Ulanga Sen

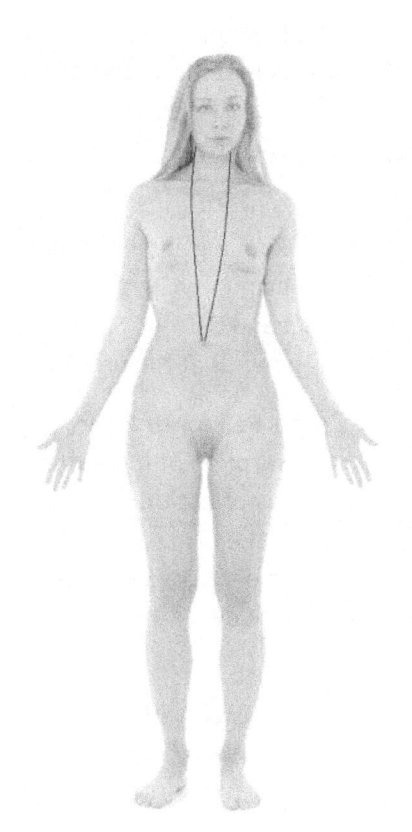

These two Sen have two alternative names in the Thai language. Lawusang is also called Chantapusang, while the Ulanga sen is also called Luchang.

Lawusang Sen originates from the navel, runs upwards on the trunk, passes next to the left ear, and ends on the temples.

Ulanga Sen follows the same path, but on the right side of the body. These two Sen control the sense of hearing.

Generally, they are used for pain on the face. They can be used for:

- earache and tinnitus (due to stress).
- any pain not due to acute inflammation (e.g. headaches).
- motion sickness.

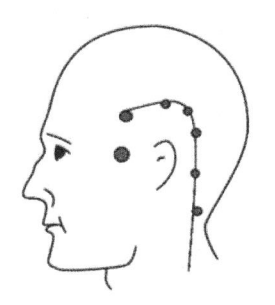

The course of Lawusang and Ulanga Sen around the ear.

10. Kitcha Sen

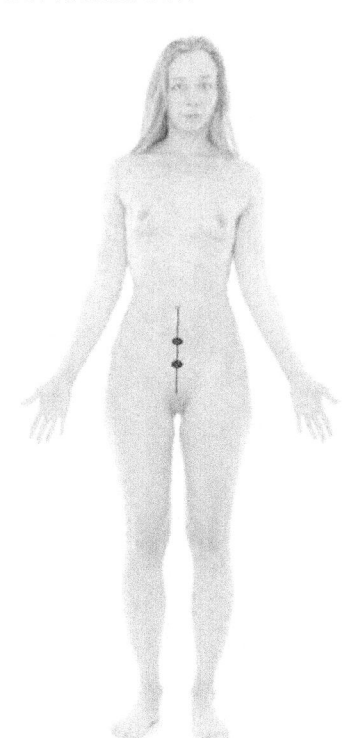

Kitcha Sen originates from the navel and descends to the genitals. In women ends on the clitoris, and is called Kitchana. In men, it reaches the end of the penis, and is called Pittakun.

Generally, it is controls sexual arousal, and reproductive capacity and function. Kitcha Sen is used mainly in cases of sexual frigidity, erectile dysfunction, and also for disorders of the female reproductive system.

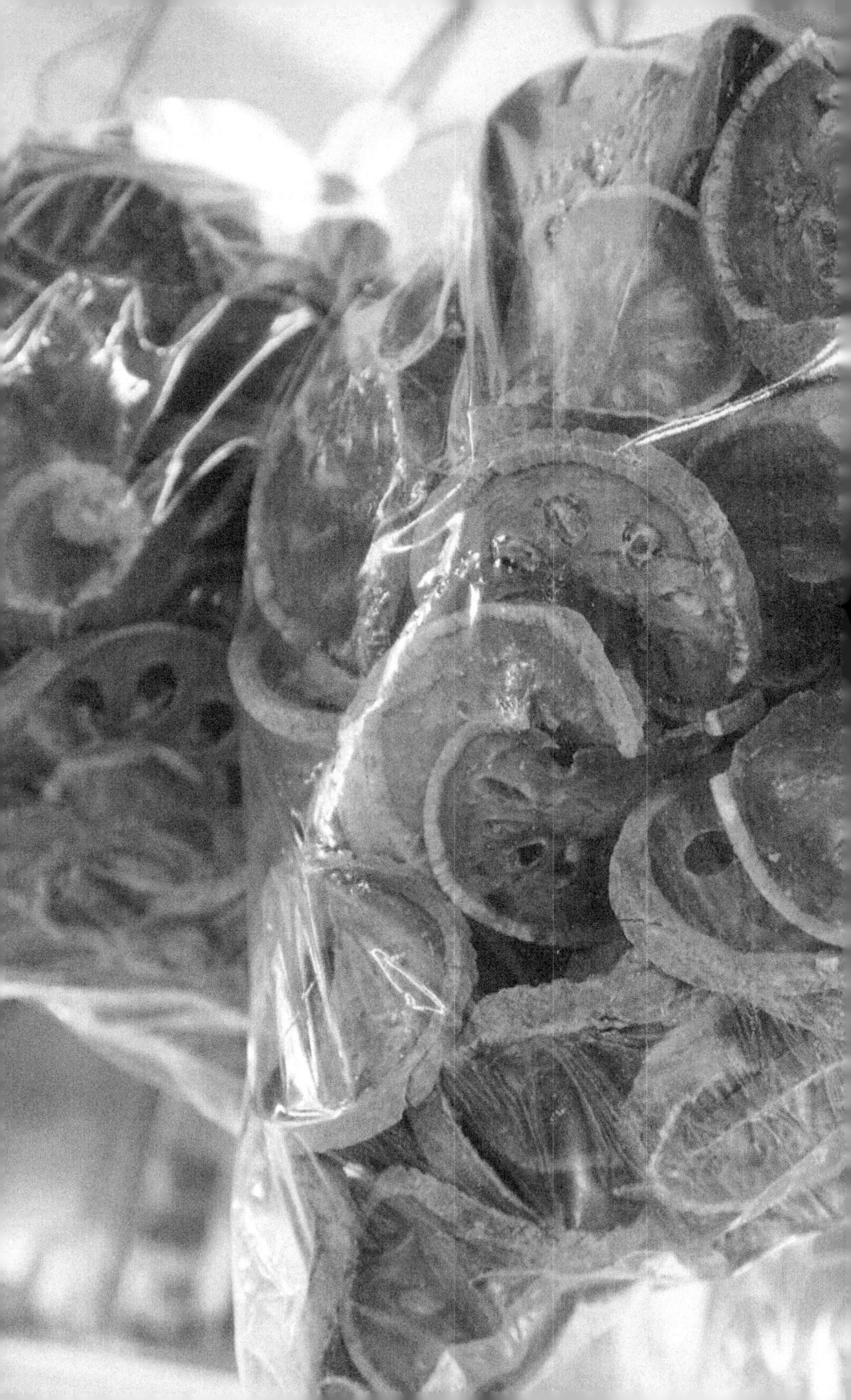

Foraging for herbs

It is possible to forage some herbs that are suitable for the herbal packs. I am sure that any urban herbalist will identify easily eucalyptus trees. Other herbs that can be harvested and identified easily include chamomile, calendula, mint and willow.

Here are some simple rules for sustainable and safe foraging:

1. **Collect only plants you are able to identify accurately**. The best way to learn this, is to attend "herb walks" with qualified instructors. Be aware of any poisonous lookalikes.

2. **Never collect threatened or endangered herbs**. E.g., in many areas of Greece it is forbidden to harvest any species from the Orchidaceae, Liliaceae and Paeoniaceae families, while it is not allowed to collect anything from the Natura network (a network of nature protection areas in the territory of the European Union). Educate yourself about the rules and the laws of your area.

3. **Avoid places subjected to pollution**. It is recommended to harvest plants that grow at least 50 meters away from roadsides, industrial buildings and agricultural land or gardens that may be sprayed with pesticides and other toxic substances. If you suspect that a plant may be contaminated, do not collect it.

4. **Harvest responsibly**. Do not uproot plants. Collect only the ¼ of the herb you are interested in, that grows in the area, so that the ecosystem balances will be maintained. Never gather more than what you really need.

5. **Respect properties**. Never trespass private properties.

These are the tools you will need:

- Bags or baskets.
- A sharp knife, pruner, and / or scissors.
- Hat, hiking clothes, rain jacket and gloves (some plants are thorny).

Enjoy foraging – it is always very satisfying to make herbal packs with plants you have collected yourself!

34. Solanum torvum, known as makhuea phuang in Thai and wild eggplant in English, growing wild in Doi Inthanon National Park in Northern Thailand. It is a plant foraged sustainably by the hill tribes that inhabit the area.

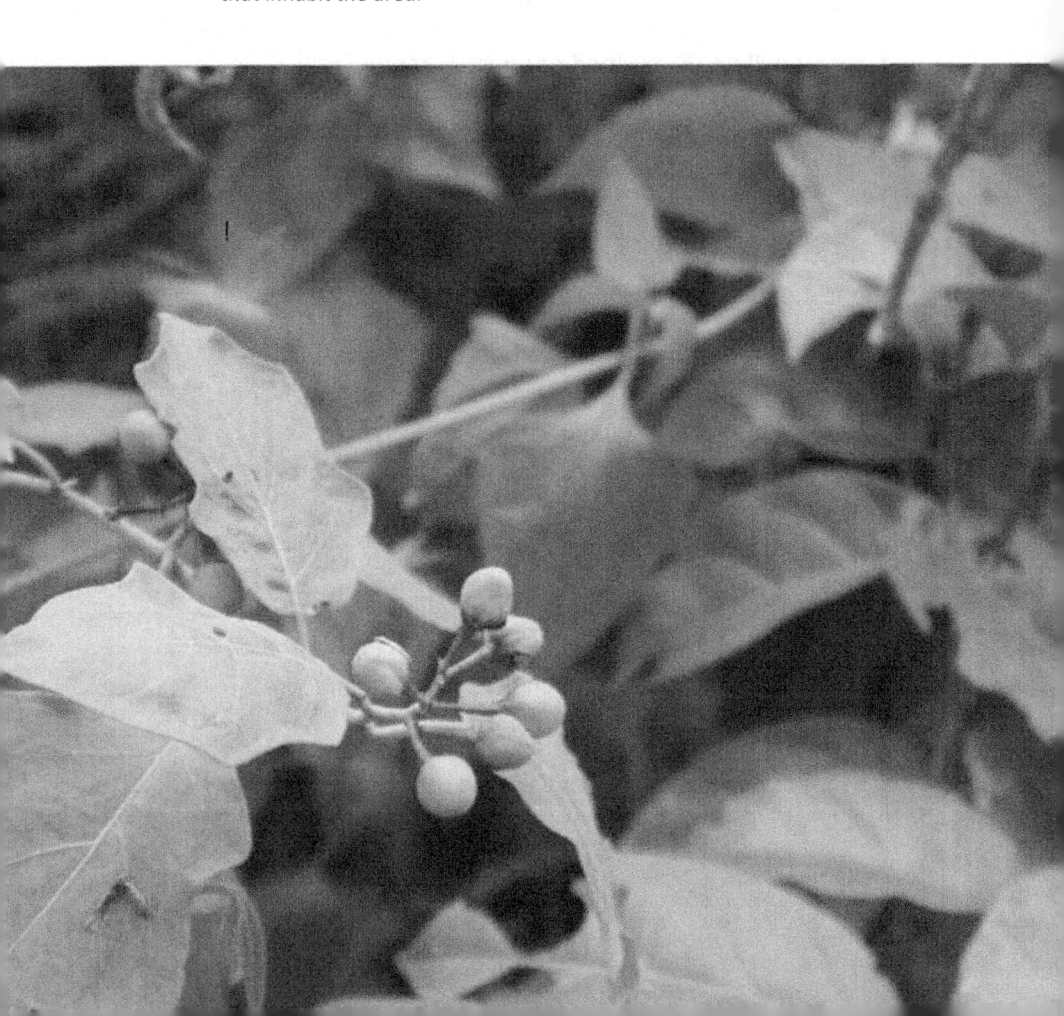

How to store herbs and herbal balls

First of all, you can use fresh herbs in your herbal balls. In that case, you do not have to dry or store anything. Of course, you have to dispose the herbal material after your treatment, as it will not last (well, it may last 2-3 days in the fridge, if you are using them at home).

If you buy dried herbs, store them in airtight glass containers, preferably dark-colored to prevent oxidation. Herbs can be stored up to six months, but powdered herbs should be discarded after two months. Store herbs in a dark, cool and dry spot.

If you forage for herbs, you should dry them before storage. Spread them on a flat surface (like a large baking tray or a rack) and turn them frequently to ensure even drying.

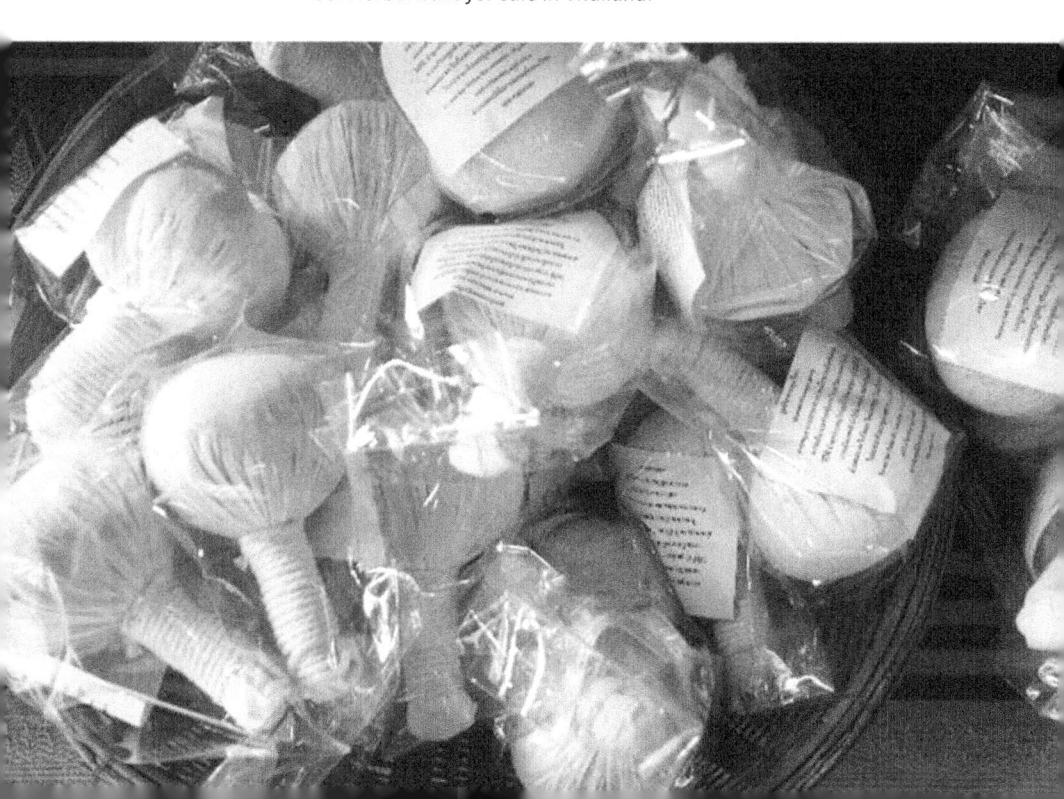

35. Herbal balls for sale in Thailand.

Another option is to tie the herbs into small bunches and hang them to dry. Leaves should face downward, and the bunches should be loose, in order to prevent mold formation.

Herbs should be completely dry and ready for storage within ten days, if you apply one of these "natural" methods of drying.

Of course, you can use a dehydrator or an oven to speed up the process.

How to store herbal balls

If your herbal balls contain dried herbs, they can be stored for at least six months. Well, they will not go mouldy after that, but the herbs will have lost their potency. Store them either in airtight containers, or in sealed plastic bags.

If you plan to store herbal balls in the fridge, they should also be placed in a sealed bag or an airtight container, otherwise their scent will saturate anything that exists in the fridge. I have eaten camphor-scented cheese, and believe me, it did not taste nice.

Epilogue

I hope you liked this book. Please have in mind that it is a small budget production, and it was made mostly by one person – me!

Most of these photos were shot in my trips in Northern Thailand, the ultimate land of herbal balls!

May these techniques be useful for your practice, your friends and your family. If you have not attended a course on herbal packs or herbal massage, I hope it will inspire you to do it.

Keep making herbal compresses and drink looots of tea!

36. Bombax ceiba, known as dok niew in Thailand. It is used both in the Thai medical tradition, and in Thai cuisine.

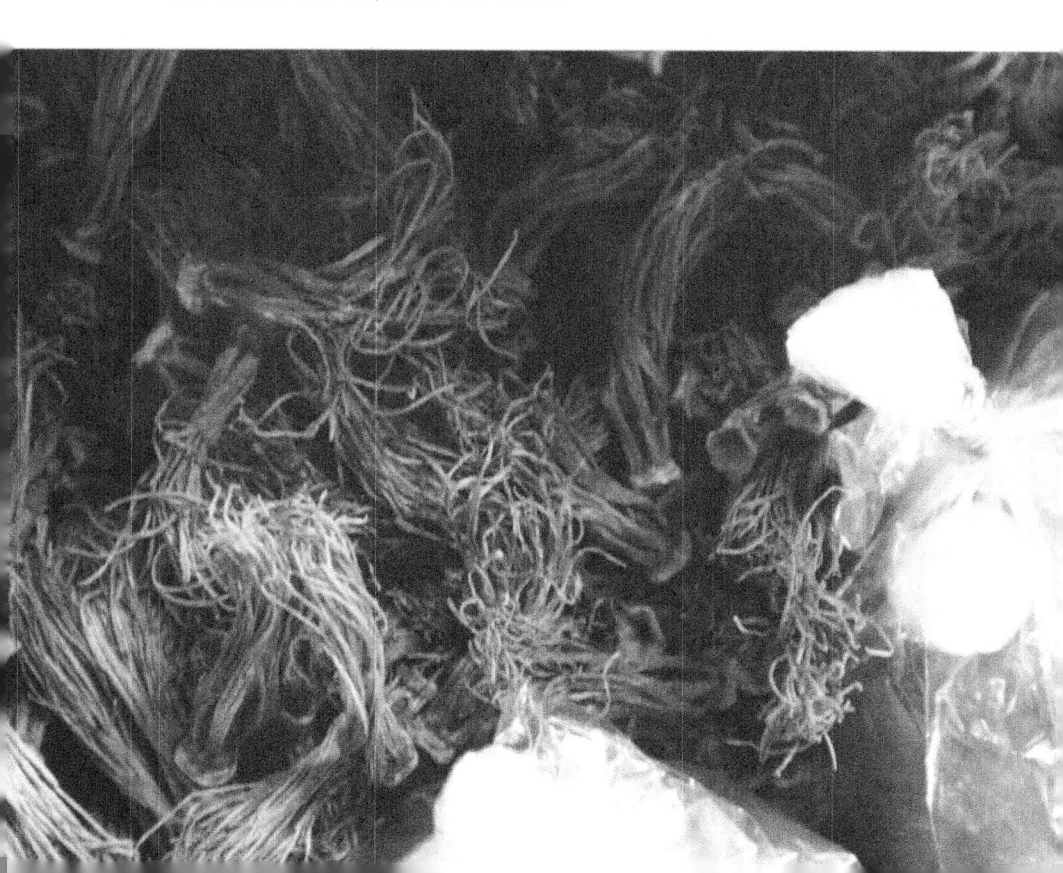

About the author

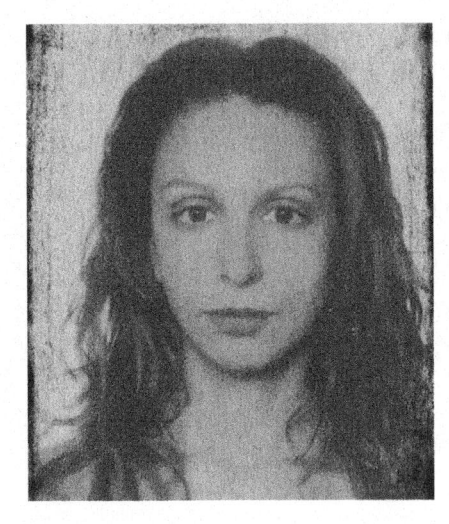

My name is Elefteria Mantzorou. I was born in Athens, Greece. From my childhood I felt attracted to herbal medicine and alternative treatments.

Disregarding any common sense, and following the flow of events without any conscious decisions, I found myself in Thailand many times. There, I studied Thai Massage, Thai Foot Massage & Thai Herbal Compress at the Old Medicine Hospital, and at the school of the unforgettable Mama Lek and her son Jack Chaiya. I also met personally Tai Chi instructor, Tew Bunnag.

For several years I lived as a backpacker. I went to many places in Europe and Asia, working as a volunteer, studying, staying in ashrams, or simply traveling. I worked as a volunteer in wildlife sanctuaries, and have treated countless wild animals. In these sanctuaries, I also worked as a surgeon's assistant.

Another experience that has remained indelible in my memory is my acquaintance with Masanobu Fukuoka and natural farming, as I had volunteered in one of his projects in Greece.

In between my trips, I studied alternative medicine (aromatherapy, herbal medicine, Swedish massage and anatomy, physiology and pathology) and was certified as a medical translator. I also attended courses on osteopathy. I started teaching in 2004, and since then I have trained hundreds of people.

In 2013 I opened my own school, FLOW, in a quiet neighborhood of Athens. Well, until I start travelling again, you might find me somewhere here:

FLOW - Wellness & Training
8, Milona str., 11363 Athens
Website: jointheflow.weebly.com

Facebook: Flow – Wellness and Training
Instagram: @FlowAthens
YouTube: Flow – Wellness and Training

Newsletter: https://bit.ly/2lBLB1t

Be always well!

Other works

You can see the other books I have published in Amazon here: amazon.com/author/elefteriamantzorou

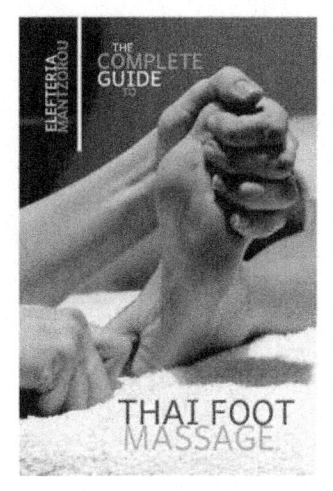

This book contains many techniques for the foot, the ankle and the lower leg, with detailed instructions.

Includes massage techniques with wooden reflexology tools.

Check out also the DVD "Thai Foot Massage", which includes the techniques of this book.

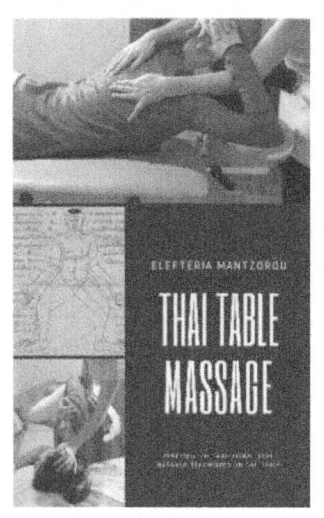

Learn to apply the traditional Thai Massage techniques on the massage table.

Take your massage therapy skills to the next level with Thai mobilizations.

The material of this book is also available in the DVD "Thai Table Massage", which is sold separately by Amazon.

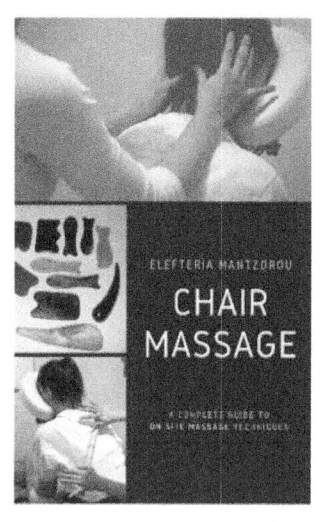

Master On Site - chair massage - techniques. Includes work with gua sha and bamboo tools.

The material of this book is also available in a DVD, which is sold separately by Amazon: "Professional Chair Massage".

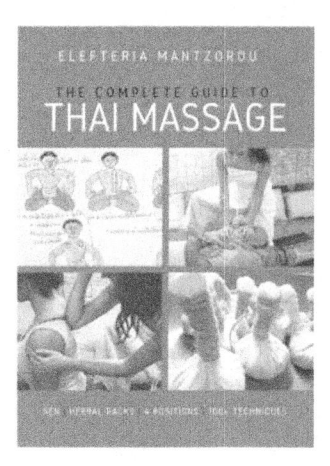

The Complete Guide to Traditional Thai Massage contains valuable information about this ancient, sacred form of bodywork. Includes sections on Sip Sen.

This book is indispensable for the serious massage therapist, as well as for anyone who studies any form of bodywork. It will be also useful for those who simply wish to learn some massage techniques in order to apply them to family members and friends.

The material of this book is also available in a DVD, which is sold separately from Amazon, as "The Complete Guide to Thai Massage".

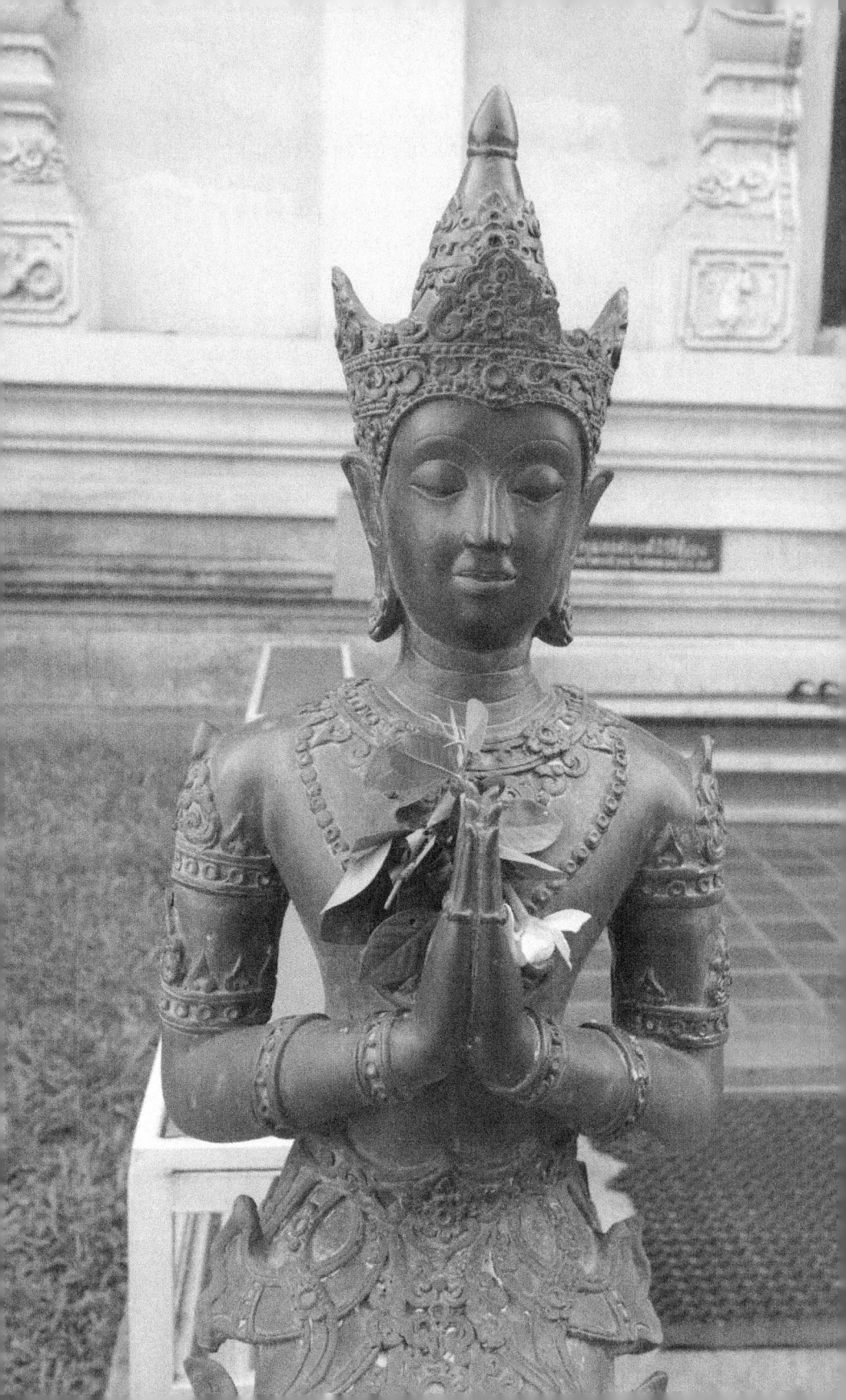

Credits

All photos (except the ones mentioned below) constitute copyrighted property of Elefteria Mantzorou. Their non-authorized use will be persecuted.

The herbal illustrations in the sections that describe the medicinal properties of herbs are in the public domain. The anatomy plates are from Gray's Anatomy, and are also in the public domain. Photos of galangal on pages 59, 60 and 61 are taken from Wikipedia commons. The rice photo on page 80 is in the public domain, and was taken from Pixabay.

Design, text and artwork by Elefteria Mantzorou.

References

[i] Traditional Herbal Medicine in Northern Thailand, Viggo Brun & Trond Schumacher.

[ii] Source: Wikipedia.org

[iii] Effect of Warm Compress and Deep Breathing Exercise on the Reduction of Primary Dysmenorrhea, Precilia Mustika Dini Kharisma, Wahyuni - Study Program of Physiotherapy, Universitas Muhammadiyah, Surakarta

[iv] Teerapon Dhippayom, Chuenjid Kongkaew, Nathorn Chaiyakunapruk, et al., "Clinical Effects of Thai Herbal Compress: A Systematic Review and Meta-Analysis," Evidence-Based Complementary and Alternative Medicine, vol. 2015, Article ID 942378, 14 pages, 2015. https://doi.org/10.1155/2015/942378.

[v] C. Trainapakul, M. Chaiyawattana, W. Kanavitoon et al., "Effect of milk ejection performance of postpartum mothers after breasts massage and compression with mini hot bag and herbal compress," Journal of Nursing and Education, vol. 3, pp. 75–91, 2010.

[vi] S. Iampornchai, S. Poopong, S. Nongbuadee et al., "Court-type traditional Thai massage and hot herbal compress: effectiveness in relieving early postpartum backache," Journal of Thai Traditional & Alternative Medicine, vol. 7, pp. 181–188, 2009.

[vii] Image taken from Wikipedia.org

[viii] Source: Wikipedia.org

[ix] Zegeye, Haileab. (2010). Environmental and Socio-economic Implications of Eucalyptus in Ethiopia.

[x] Galeotti, N.; Mannelli, L. D. C.; Mazzanti, G.; Bartolini, A.; Ghelardini, C.; Di Cesare, Mannelli (2002). "Menthol: a natural analgesic compound".

[xi] Hewlings SJ, Kalman DS. Curcumin: A Review of Its' Effects on Human Health. Foods. 2017;6(10):92. Published 2017 Oct 22. doi:10.3390/foods6100092

[xii] Hypoglycemic Activity of Ruellia tuberosa Linn (Acanthaceae) in Normal and Alloxan-Induced Diabetic Rabbits, Article 8,

Volume 7, Issue 2, Spring 2011, Page 107-115, Durre Shahwar et al.
[xiii] Source: Wikipedia.org
[xiv] Photo and text taken from Wikipedia.
[xv] http://www.stuartxchange.org/Sambong.html
[xvi] Source: Wikipedia.org
[xvii] Parente, Leila Maria Leal et al. "Wound Healing and Anti-Inflammatory Effect in Animal Models of Calendula officinalis L. Growing in Brazil." Evidence-based complementary and alternative medicine : eCAM vol. 2012 (2012): 375671. doi:10.1155/2012/375671
[xviii] Native American Ehnobotany Database. http://naeb.brit.org
[xix] Boonruab J, Damjuti W, Niempoog S, Pattaraarchachai J. Effectiveness of hot herbal compress versus topical diclofenac in treating patients with myofascial pain syndrome. J Tradit Complement Med. 2018;9(2):163–167. Published 2018 Jun 1. doi:10.1016/j.jtcme.2018.05.004.

Made in the USA
Coppell, TX
21 May 2023